The Reaper's Compromise:

How Payers, Policy-Makers, and Patients Wreck Health Care

By

Thorsten O'Shaughnessy

The Reaper's Compromise: How Payers, Policy-Makers, and Patients Wreck Health Care by Thorsten O'Shaughnessy

Published by Thorsten O'Shaughnessy

www.thereaperscompromise.wordpress.com

Cover by Margaret Feinheimer

"Our healthcare system is broken." One can scarcely turn on the television, listen to the radio, or even engage in casual conversation with friends and neighbors without someone uttering this very simple sentence. While certainly very few would disagree, a deeper analysis of the rationale behind such an assertion reveals a wide diversity of opinions.

The physician might claim the system is broken because of extreme levels of paperwork or declining compensation. The patient will root his or her dissatisfaction with the size of their bill. An executive will rail against increasing levels of regulation. Politicians will demonize anyone or anything that could stir popular opinion to help them win re-election. Each of these groups will be considering the "brokenness" of the system from their own very understandable perspectives. However, very few will be able to explain why paperwork has increased, why bills are higher, or the substance of the healthcare policies they claim to support or condemn.

This cannot be overstated. The overwhelming majority of persons who discuss healthcare matters have very little idea what they are talking about. If they do, they are often beholden to particular ideological or political theories that override their common sense and direct them to solutions that only make the problem worse. After all, for the political animal, results are secondary to winning, and the service to the public gives way to the service of power.

Now, I can understand if you read those lines and think "If that's the case, why should I listen to anything that anyone says, including this book?" That is a perfectly reasonable reaction to have. Allow me to explain why this book might be of more value than others.

I came into healthcare and worked my way up to an executive level position. The experience was very much like the Kubler-Ross Five Stages of Grief.[1] At first, I was in utter disbelief that those charged with running our healthcare system could be so obtuse in dealing with such grave matters. Disbelief gave way to anger, as I realized that incompetence could not explain the dangerous nature of their actions. No, there was intent as well. Bargaining took the form of trying to reason with myself that there really was no better system and that we had to live with what we had. Depression came from

---

[1] Elisabeth Kubler-Ross was a Swiss-American psychiatrist whose work *On Death and Dying* (1969) claimed that patients who received a terminally ill diagnosis typically undergo five stages of grief in coming to grips with their impending death: denial, anger, bargaining, depression and acceptance.

realizing that political figures and insurers were bent on ever more destructive measures and that nobody was even remotely mobilized or in a position to stop them.[2]

As I dealt more and more with policy makers, payers, and other organs of the healthcare system, it became clear that much of what was done at various levels of government was done in order to exploit the complexity of the healthcare system and most citizens' lack of knowledge. To be clear, "most citizens" here includes highly educated individuals, including physicians. I have a great working relationship with the physicians at my facility, but I can tell you almost all of them will admit to complete ignorance over real healthcare regulations and payment structures. Even physician members of Congress (along with most other members of Congress) demonstrate a shocking lack of knowledge about what they are doing with the subject of healthcare.

If this seems outrageous to you, consider the words of economics professor Jonathan Gruber of the Massachusetts Institute of Technology. Professor Gruber was heavily involved in Massachusetts's re-design of

---

[2] More than anything else, I suppose you could say this book is a work of acceptance.

their state's healthcare system in 2006, and more famously as a high-level consultant in the drafting of the Patient Protection and Affordable Care Act[3] in 2009 and 2010. In a moment of refreshing honesty in 2013, Professor Gruber made the following comments regarding the passage of the law:

> *This bill was written in a tortured way to make sure [the Congressional Budget Office] did not score the mandate as taxes. If CBO scored the mandate as taxes, the bill dies. OK? So it's written to do that. In terms of risk-rated subsidies, if you had a law which said healthy people are going to pay in — you made explicit that healthy people pay in and sick people get money — it would not have passed. OK?* **Lack of transparency is a huge political advantage. And**

<blockquote>

basically, call it the stupidity of the American voter or whatever, but basically that was really, really critical to get the thing to pass. Look, I wish ... we could make it all transparent, but I'd rather have this law than not.[4]

</blockquote>

Regardless of your political persuasion, please do not take these words as the standard pundit approach of "Democrat BAD...Republican GOOD!" I seek to demonstrate here that they are both bad, usually because they have very little idea of what they are saying and therefore wind up parroting buzzwords about which their knowledge is a mile wide and half an inch deep.

To refer back to the issue of my own credibility, I can only say that I will be honest with you. I am not going to offer much in the way of answers or solutions because they are beyond any one person or government body. My

---

[4] https://www.youtube.com/watch?v=Adrdmmh7bMo at the 00:10 mark. The video also features an additional example of Professor Gruber commenting on how American voters are "too stupid to know the difference" between having their own taxes raised vs. having their insurance company taxed and passing the cost of a tax onto the insured in the form of a higher price. He also comments that this provision of the ACA was "a very clever basic exploitation of the lack of economic understanding of the American voter."

goal in writing this is to try and illustrate why healthcare is broken and why no political or medical messiah is going to be able to fix it. Ultimately, our society has made a deal with Death, to the extent that numbers, dollar signs, and convenience have become the priorities over and above life itself. I also beg your pardon on what might be seen as an overuse of quotes and citations. I have found in my attempts to explain these matters to people that they do not readily believe me. This has led me to excessively document the points I'm trying to make. Hopefully, you will find this helpful rather than annoying.

There is one last item to address. No, my name is not Thorsten O'Shaughnessy. I am certain to draw much anger in writing under a pseudonym. I ask for your sympathy in doing so. As we will discuss in these pages, the healthcare system is governed by a large mass of politicians, bureaucrats, and corporate interests, and the lines between these parties blur very easily. I still work in healthcare. I have a wife and a family. I have co-workers who shed an extreme amount of blood, sweat, and tears while toiling over the care of the sick and infirm. The governing interests of healthcare will not like this book. If it draws their attention, they will attempt to retaliate against me for writing it. If I've learned any lesson from these years in this industry, it is that anyone trying to raise real understanding of these matters or protesting the system status quo will be ruthlessly persecuted to the point of having their entire organization's sustainability jeopardized. For that reason, I must and will remain anonymous, as will the sources of my discussions and anecdotes.

I hope that this explanation suffices. I hope this work is helpful to you.

Thank you for your interest in the truth.

Chapter 1: Defining Our Terms

Explaining the scope of our nation's healthcare problems requires knowledge of some of the basic terminology associated with the topic. I present the following description of terms and abbreviations here in order to make the discussion in the upcoming pages easier to follow. If you have a working knowledge of the structure of our healthcare system, you might find these items simple or redundant, but it seemed valuable to include for the many who might not.

Much of national healthcare policy is determined by the **Department of Health and Human Services (HHS).** The head of HHS is part of the President's Cabinet and is nominated to that position by the President for confirmation by the Senate. The current Secretary of HHS is Alex Azar, who previously served as the President of the US Division of Eli Lilly & Co., a large pharmaceutical company. The Secretary has broad executive power to propose and adopt rules and regulations for healthcare in the US. These rules and regulations have the force of law, despite not having to pass before Congress or be signed by the President.

The most prominent sub-unit of the Department of Health and Human Services is the **Centers for Medicare and Medicaid (CMS)**. As its name suggests, CMS is charged with administering the Medicare and Medicaid programs (which we will describe in a bit). As part of that responsibility, it also regulates hospitals, nursing homes, and other healthcare facilities. It has ten regional offices scattered throughout the United States. It is led by an Administrator, with the current Administrator being Seema Verma, a healthcare policy consultant who served as the primary lead on Medicaid reform in Indiana under Governors Mitch Daniels and Mike Pence. Like Mr. Azar, Ms. Verma has executive rule-making authority over the various organizations that come under the CMS umbrella.

Medicare is the federally funded program meant to pay for the health care of eligible elderly or disabled Americans. It essentially amounts to an insurance program for those over the age of 65 who have been legal residents for over five years. It also covers younger individuals who receive Social Security Disability benefits or have certain specific illnesses, such as Lou Gherig's Disease. Medicare was signed into law by President Lyndon Johnson in 1965. Over the years, Medicare coverage has expanded and is now divided up into four parts:

1. Part A - This is the Medicare benefit that pays for hospice care, inpatient stays in a hospital, or rehabilitation services in a skilled nursing facility (SNF) such as a nursing home. As we will see later, Medicare Part A is subject to deductibles and coinsurance, as well as a myriad of rules as to when and how the coverage actually applies. Part A also has a premium structure, but the premiums are waived for those eligible parties who have paid Medicare taxes for ten years and those in some of the aforementioned disability/illness categories.

2. Part B - Part B benefits generally apply to outpatient encounters such as visits to the doctor, imaging (x-rays, MRIs, etc.), lab tests, and so forth. Part B also pays for observation stays in a hospital, but we will go into greater detail about that later. Part B has its own deductible, copay, and coinsurance structure. In addition, there is typically a premium of $135.50 per month.[5] There is no waiver provision like with Part A. Moreover, there are

---

[5] There is a "hold harmless" provision for individuals when an increase in their monthly Social Security benefit does not cover the cost of their Part B premium. As a result, this is not a certainty.

certain additional taxes for funding Part B that fall on those making more than $85,000 per year.

3. Part C - This is a reference to Medicare Managed Care, also known as Medicare Advantage. Originating in 1997 in a law signed by President Bill Clinton, Part C plans involve a Medicare recipient opting to have a private insurance company, known as a managed care organization (MCO), manage their Medicare benefits. The MCO typically works in the same fashion as an HMO. The federal government, through CMS, provides them with a set payment per Medicare beneficiary they have as an enrollee. The MCO then tries to find ways to keep their enrollees so healthy that they do not require any payments to be made for health care services. If the MCO is successful in holding down the costs of the patient's care, they make a surplus on their government payments.

For example, if Joe is on a Medicare Advantage plan, and the plan receives $1,000 per month to pay for Joe's health care, the plan will try to make sure that Joe is so healthy that only $500 will need to be spent on Joe's going to the doctor, labs, and so forth. At the end of the month, having only spent $500 in taking care of Joe, the plan pockets the remaining $500 from the CMS payment. In theory, this is how the system should work. As we shall see, the true practice is something entirely different.

4. Part D - This is more commonly known as the "prescription drug benefit." Taking effect in 2006, Part D was initially signed into law by President George W. Bush. The Part D benefit is administered entirely by private insurers and pharmacy benefit managers under guidelines set by CMS. There is no single "Part D" plan, as they vary widely depending upon what the recipient selects to meet their needs.

Finally, it should be mentioned that individuals may be eligible for benefits under both Medicare and Medicaid. These are called **dual eligibles**."

Medicare Administrative Contractors (MACs) are defined as "a private health care insurer that has been awarded a geographic jurisdiction to process Medicare Part A and Part B (A/B) medical claims or Durable

Medical Equipment (DME) claims for Medicare Fee-For-Service (FFS) beneficiaries."[6] Basically, they are private companies that Medicare uses to outsource its responsibility for Medicare payments. This ranges from just paying bills from providers to making Local Coverage Determinations (LCDs), which are decisions on whether or not Medicare will cover a particular service. It's commonly thought that Medicare coverage is uniform throughout the country. This is not the case, as an LCD in Washington state might allow coverage (and therefore payment) of a certain type of surgery or medical device. That same procedure might not be covered in Mississippi due to the MAC in that region issuing a contrary LCD.

Most providers would likely tell you that MACs operate under almost zero levels of accountability. I spoke to several who told stories of their billing numbers being deactivated or unexplained delays in payment. St. Anthony's Hospital in Houston, Texas could not even make payroll and eventually went bankrupt allegedly because of the incompetence of its MAC.[7] The Texas Hospital Association was clear that St. Anthony's problems were not an isolated event, saying, "they are

---

[6] https://www.cms.gov/Medicare/Medicare-Contracting/Medicare-Administrative-Contractors/What-is-a-MAC.html
[7] https://abc13.com/archive/9372756/

familiar with complaints like this one regarding the Medicare payment facilitator, and a representative told us smaller community hospitals like this one are in similar situations." While St. Anthony's closed down, Novitas, the MAC in question, retains its contract with CMS.[8]

For what it's worth, I am unaware of how the MAC structure would work under some of the existing single payer or Medicare-for-All proposals. Part of the appeal behind such proposals is to reduce administrative burden and costs, but I'm unsure if this includes absorbing the MAC functions into a purely public entity.

Medicaid is the joint federal and state insurance program for low income individuals. Like Medicare, it was passed into law during the Johnson administration. State Medicaid plans may vary in their benefit structure and coverage decisions, with oversight from CMS. The program is funded through a state-federal matching program. States put up a certain amount of funding, with those state dollars drawing down federal dollars, with the amount determined by the Federal Matching Percentage (FMAP) formula. Under the ACA, Medicaid eligibility was significantly expanded to allow coverage for those

---

[8] I was unsuccessful in contacting any C-Suite employees from St. Anthony's for more specific details. I also did not find a response from Novitas other than the pablum quoted in the article above.

with income up to 133% of the poverty level, including previously ineligible populations, such as single males without children. In doing so, the federal government offered to pay 100% of the initial cost to those newly-enrolled individuals, with that amount eventually tapering down to 90% in 2020. As of now, 37 states have expanded their Medicaid programs to this level.

Unlike Medicare, Medicaid often has no copays, no deductibles, and no coinsurance. Some states have added proof of work requirements, modest copays (say, $3), and other factors to attempt to regulate eligibility and utilization of services. To implement such variations, the state must obtain permission from CMS.

Medicaid also typically has significantly lower payment rates than Medicare or commercial insurance. This means that a physician who sees a Medicaid patient in their office will likely be paid much lower than they would be for providing the same service to a Medicare or Aetna patient. Since the payments are so low, many health care providers do not accept Medicaid patients for their services. This creates a large problem for Medicaid enrollees, as they frequently cannot find a local provider to treat them, forcing them to travel long distances or endure long wait times for their care.[9]

Both Medicare and Medicaid tend to operate under a **fee-for-service** (FFS) model. This is the sort of payment structure used in most industries wherein a service is provided (such as a doctor visit or surgery or MRI scan) and a fee is charged for that service being rendered. While one would not usually think that this is problematic, especially given that most countries in the world work on an FFS system, it is frequently demonized as the root of all of our healthcare problems.[10] Criticisms of FFS are grounded largely in the idea that physicians and other health care providers tend to be unethical or insecure. They therefore order lots and lots of worthless tests or perform unnecessary surgery because this means they will either be (a) paid more for the tests/surgery or (b) protected from potential lawsuits because the patients have been given such a thorough work-up. This low view of physicians is highly ingrained in the healthcare bureaucracy and drives many of their decisions, as we shall see.

---

[9] You can visit https://physiciansfoundation.org/wp-content/uploads/2018/09/physicians-survey-results-final-2018.pdf for a 2018 study on what percentages of doctors will accept Medicare and Medicaid, among other interesting physician practice information.

[10] For a brief description of this perspective, see this article from *The Atlantic*: https://www.theatlantic.com/health/archive/2012/05/moving-away-from-fee-for-service/256755/

Capitation systems of payment are the most frequent alternative to FFS. In a capitated system, the health care provider is given a single payment for a patient and then expected to tend to all of the patient's health care needs from the proceeds of that single payment. For example, in a surgical setting, a surgeon might be paid $1,000 for taking out a person's appendix, and this payment is meant to compensate that surgeon for the surgery, the follow-up office visit, and any other incidents related to the operation.

On a grander scale, capitation takes the form of physicians (usually in primary care) being paid a flat rate for each patient they have enrolled in their service. In this case, a physician might be paid $500 a month per patient. That $500 is meant to take care of every visit to that physician's office and every test they might receive while there. There are other examples[11], but just keep in mind that capitation essentially means handing a health care provider some money and then expecting them to take care of a patient's needs based on that.

Capitation is, more than anything, a process of shifting risk from the health care payer (Medicare,

---

[11] See the article in n. 10 for a few. While The Atlantic doesn't call them all "capitation," they are variations on the same theme.

Medicaid, commercial insurance, etc.) to the entity charged with delivering the health care service (the physician, the hospital, etc.). *In a practical sense, it means that payments for health care services go from a provider being paid to treat and help sick people to their being paid not to treat and help sick people.* After all, the sicker the patients are, the more in need of services they will be. The more in need of services they are, the more it will cost a provider to take care of them. The more it costs a provider to take care of them, then the more those costs eat into the flat capitated amount of money the provider was given to care for the patient. The decision faced by the provider is then whether or not they actually want to take care of sicker patients, or, if they do take care of sicker patients, how to not go broke while still delivering the care the patient needs.[12]

This is to provide a foundation of some basic definitions. It is not remotely exhaustive. As new terms are introduced throughout the coming chapters, we will elaborate on their meanings to the greatest extent practical.[13]

---

[12] I'm well aware of the notion that many consider capitation as "being paid for keeping the patients well" rather than how I've described it above. The reality is that "keeping patients well" often, even usually, has absolutely nothing to do with a provider's treatment.

[13] In the interim, for additional terms related to insurance coverage, please visit this link to view the CMS glossary: https://www.cms.gov/CCIIO/Resources/Files/Downloads/uniform-glossary-final.pdf

Chapter 2: The Nature of the Compromise

I mentioned in the Introduction that our society has made a deal with Death, hence the title of this work. An analysis of the deal begins in 1994 with Dr. William Kissick's recognition of what he termed "the Iron Triangle of Health Care."[14] Dr. Kissick was a well-known professor at Yale, having obtained his BS, MD, MPH, and PhD degrees from there. The Iron Triangle consisted of three elements: cost, access, and quality. These three elements compete for resources. Generally speaking, for example, increasing quality will result in higher costs and lower access, while decreasing costs will result in lower quality and access, and so on. Solving this dilemma was ostensibly the primary goal of healthcare policy makers for decades, even if the problem hadn't been depicted in this manner. It continued to be the policy framework for years thereafter, with the focus of problem-solving focusing on ways to increase access and quality, while decreasing costs.

As time rolled by, there continued to be much clamoring about cost and quality. How many times have

---

[14] Dr. William Kissick, *Medicine's Dilemmas: Infinite Needs Versus Finite Resources*, Yale University Press (1994).

you tuned in to hear a talking head on a news network excoriating healthcare in the United States for delivering low quality at a high cost? I'm guessing it's quite frequently. Notice that access is typically not part of the conversation now. As a point of concern, its status has been in decline for some time.

Consider the standard admonitions from the average politician regarding healthcare. There is a massive amount of ink spilled and verbal diarrhea about how to help people pay for health care. The reforms of the ACA were primarily geared towards finding coverage for the uninsured, whether by expanding Medicaid or by providing them with a commercial plan purchased off of an insurance exchange. You rarely heard anyone inquire about whether or not these newly covered patients would actually be able to receive care from a willing provider, either from a primary care or specialist perspective.

The deletion of "access" from the policy vocabulary was formalized in 2007 by Dr. Don Berwick, a Harvard-educated pediatrician who briefly served as the head of CMS, and the Institute for Healthcare Improvement, a not-for-profit based in Cambridge, Massachusetts. Instead of speaking of the Iron Triangle of access/cost/quality, the new focus is what is known as the

Triple Aim. The Triple Aim is made up of cost, population (as opposed to individual) health outcomes, and patient experience. Whether deliberate or not, this change in verbiage has largely (and subtly) excised the nature of health care access from our collective political discussion.

This is not to say that Dr. Berwick & Co. flipped a switch, changing the conversation overnight. They merely gave a linguistic framework to decisions that were already underway; namely, decisions that pushed access to the lowest priority of the access/cost/quality hierarchy, ignoring the simple fact that individuals who cannot access the healthcare system will naturally have worse health outcomes. They will, however, eventually have lower costs. If there is restricted access to the system, how can they generate a bill for services? Moreover, if they experience higher mortality rates and die off quicker, they are permanently off of the government's books and no longer a driver of costs.

From a purely anecdotal point of view, I can tell you that I have been to dozens of conferences where the Triple Aim has been discussed. Access is not on the agenda. When presenters are asked about access, they tend to obfuscate by claiming that devoting resources to population health will solve the access problem. This raises two issues. First, it admits that the Triple Aim prioritizes groups over individuals, with the priority being on larger groups who, of course, have higher levels of cost to control and are therefore more important to the government as a payer. Second, in practical application, it has very little to do with what health care providers face day in and day out due to factors utterly out of their control.

The end result of all of this is that payers, specifically government payers, are now crafting healthcare policies with the explicit concentration being almost exclusively on cost but dressed up in flowery language about higher quality. These strategies almost always entail some sort of damage to health care access, with more and more providers considering limiting their engagement with patients enrolled with these programs. This is the government's compromise with The Reaper. It is willing to exchange the health and lives of its citizens for a reduction in costs and a greater level of control over the health of the masses. I must emphasize again that both of the major political parties in the United States have different rhetorical flourishes in dealing with healthcare. However, a close examination of their stated proposals almost always tends to limit patient access. We will see some of these examples in the coming pages.

As government payers pick up more and more of the healthcare costs in the United States[15], this will become a greater factor in people's lives. It won't happen overnight, to be sure. It will be by slow increments, as we have seen over the last couple of decades, and will be fueled by both political parties.

This is not a problem limited to the government. The healthcare consumer has their own lethal deal that they cling to regardless of consequences. Consider some of the following statistics.

> In a survey of 723 patient care sites by medical liability insurer The Doctors Company, 53% of respondents said referrals and scheduling follow-up

---

appointments were their top risk-management problems...
A separate review of 2,466 claims between 2007 and 2011 by The Doctors Company found that 36% of patient injuries resulted from patient factors such as noncompliance with follow-up calls and not adhering to treatment regimens.[16]

Notice that this is only tracking providers expressing risk management concerns and patients who have experienced injuries. This is not illustrative of the total numbers of noncompliant patients. Patients who do not abide by the medical advice given to them by their health care provider is its own epidemic.

Yet, patients do ignore doctor's orders, and much more frequently than physicians would care to acknowledge. In 2011, nearly

---

16

https://amednews.com/article/20130715/profession/130719980/2/

half a million admitted
patients, 1 to 2 percent, left
American hospitals "A.M.A."
— against medical advice. A
2010 Harvard Medical School
study showed that about 20
percent of first-time
prescriptions are never filled.
According to the Centers for
Disease Control and
Prevention, fewer than two of
three Americans over 50 have
received recommended
screening for colon cancer.[17]

These are staggering numbers. One in five patients
are prescribed medication but don't bother to pick up
even the first dose. Half a million patients are sick enough
to need a hospital admission and then leave even as they
are being told not to do so.

Poor medication compliance
is to blame for about 125,000
deaths per year, as well 10

---

[17] https://www.bostonglobe.com/lifestyle/health-wellness/2013/04/21/practice-why-patients-don-always-follow-orders/6HRxBeEuLf7jCk2pu7ilKP/story.html

percent of hospital and 23 percent of nursing home admissions. About 36 million U.S. adults smoke cigarettes, despite evidence that it increases the risk for lung and 17 other cancers, coronary heart disease, stroke, chronic obstructive pulmonary disease (COPD) and other respiratory illnesses. Almost 90 percent people living with type 2 diabetes are overweight or obese. Just a small amount of weight loss could decrease the amount of medication needed to keep blood sugar within a healthy range.

When these patients seek care, they are often sicker and require more intense and expensive treatment. Research shows patients who do not take medications as prescribed by their doctors cost the U.S. health care system about $290 billion in avoidable medical spending every year. Besides those costs – about 13 percent of total health care spending – there's also $1.5 billion annually in lost patient earnings and $50 billion in lost productivity.[18]

How often do you hear about this problem in popular political rants? It's doubtful that you've ever heard it at all unless you are speaking with a health care provider still in the trenches. It's certainly bad form to criticize potential voters, so politicians will keep silent on how much of our healthcare brokenness is directly related to patients' reluctance to follow instructions. In reality, the problem is much worse than what is illustrated in these quotes.

For example, in our experience in the facility where I work, we made an effort to schedule every patient

____

[18]

http://www.makingthehealthcaresystemwork.com/2017/09/27/igno
ring-doctors-orders-the-high-cost-of-noncompliance/

who was discharged from the hospital an appointment with their primary care provider. These appointments were scheduled for three to five days after their discharge, with the patient's input and participation in picking an exact day and time. Of those patients, 42% did not show up for their visit. In order to try and resolve this problem, we engaged the services of a full-time employee whose job is to schedule appointments, contact patients to remind them of their appointments, and then reschedule if the date/time were no longer convenient. Less than 20% of those contacted re-scheduled. Even with these measures in place, the no-show rate only dropped 8%. This cost, and those like it, aren't measured in the quoted statistics. However, they do eat into the margin of a healthcare organization.

There are an infinite number of reasons why a person might not make their follow-up visit or miss their medication dose or decline to change their diet/exercise regimen. Many might chalk up these habits of noncompliance to economic factors. Perhaps the patient cannot afford their medication. This is obviously a problem, but does it explain their unwillingness to walk around the block or show up for a visit? Many facilities (such as our own) offer no-cost transportation to patients, regardless of their payer. What if a pill isn't needed at all?

> "I [the doctor] wonder sometimes why they even come to see me. I write a prescription, we talk about a game plan to get them on the path to success and then they come back in a year and we talk about it all over again because they didn't do anything I said," he says. "Or they come in and I talk to them about changing their diet and losing 10 pounds and their blood pressure would probably come down on its own. But they give you a blank look and say 'can't you just give me a pill?'"[19]

The patient, as human nature often dictates, is looking for the path of least resistance and minimal accountability.

Others suggest that the real problem is a lack of patient education and that, if providers only spent more

---

[19] Id.

time explaining to patients the severity of their illness and the consequences of noncompliance, patients would naturally respond and adhere to whatever treatment was prescribed. This is difficult to take seriously, considering the national phenomenon of smoking. The CDC estimates that 38 million Americans smoke.[20] This is in spite of labeling on the package telling the consumer that the item they are purchasing is harmful to their health. This is in spite of massive media, legal, and health campaigns, some with truly grotesque content, blaring the multiple ways in which tobacco usage can cause sickness, disfigurement, and death. Yet smoking endures.[21]

I'm reminded of a young medical student (let's call her Ivy) who was in a rotation following one of our physicians. Ivy was determined to be a family practice or internal medicine physician. Primary care was her passion, or so she thought. She engaged every patient with a thorough review of their chart and, in the case of

---

[20] https://www.cdc.gov/media/releases/2018/p0118-smoking-rates-declining.html

[21] Just one other note to reinforce the point: "About half the people who undergo kidney transplants do not adequately adhere to the regimen necessary to thwart rejection of their new organ. A 1970s study found that 43 percent of glaucoma patients refused to take the doctor-ordered measures necessary to prevent blindness, even when that refusal had already led to blindness in one eye." https://slate.com/technology/2008/03/the-mystery-of-patients-who-fail-to-follow-prescriptions.html

smokers, would always ask them why the physician had never talked to them before about quitting smoking. The typical patient response was to laugh at Ivy's zeal and inform her that, yes, the doctor had been talking to them about quitting for a long time (decades for some). After several weeks of this phenomenon repeating itself multiple times a day, along with similar reactions to her pleas that patients drink fewer soft drinks, walk for 15 minutes a day, and so forth, Ivy found herself thoroughly disillusioned. She went on to reject a primary care calling and opted for a specialty that was less oriented toward managing chronic conditions.

Do not take these comments as judgments. I'm a terrible patient and noncompliant with the majority of what my primary care providers will tell me, much to their chagrin. I readily admit that I'm part of the problem. What is that problem specifically? It is this: we, as patients and consumers of health care resources, have made our own deal with The Reaper. We are happy to trade him away years of our lives in exchange for convenience, low out-of-pocket costs, and just plain not being bothered by the strain of doing what is best for our own well-being and also that of society in general.

Perhaps you think this statement is an exaggeration. As a final example, I present the following:

> Eager to learn more about the perceived utility of daily pills, a team of researchers conducted an Internet-based study of 1,000 Americans with a mean age of 50. They asked the participants how they felt about taking a daily pill that would prevent cardiovascular disease—and how much of their life they would give up in order not to have to take a pill every day. Though about 70 percent of participants said they wouldn't trade a moment to avoid taking a pill, 21 percent said they'd trade anywhere from a week to a year of their lives. And more than 8 percent surveyed said that they would trade as many as

two years of their lives to
avoid taking a daily pill.[22]

These results were after the surveyors qualified that the pills in question would cost nothing and come with zero side effects.[23] The only thing the patient would be sacrificing was the 60 seconds or so that it would take to swallow the medication. To reiterate: one in three people who were surveyed stated that they would trade part of their lives away to avoid taking a daily pill. Almost one in ten were willing to trade away **_years_**. These are only the ones who were willing to admit it. It doesn't count those individuals who might have been too embarrassed to say so, nor does it take into consideration any who, once given such a pill, would not do so out of absent-mindedness, negligence, or apathy.

Whether people wish to acknowledge it or not, a choice has been made. When given options between health and inconvenience/costs vs. sickness and convenience/disposable income, a significant portion of

---

[22] https://www.smithsonianmag.com/smart-news/1-3-would-rather-die-early-take-daily-pill-180954141/

[23] At least one recent survey indicates that patients are unwilling to accept lower drug costs if that means the potential for fewer new drugs on the market: https://www.cnbc.com/2019/03/06/americans-want-lower-prescription-prices-but-not-fewer-drugs-survey.html.

the population has opted for the latter. In the coming pages, I hope to provide examples of how these compromises manifest themselves in policies and why providers, usually cast in the role of the villain, are fighting an uphill battle between crushing governmental regulations and reimbursement cuts meant to kill patient access, commercial insurance companies looking out for shareholder interests, and patient indifference which, in the era of providers taking on greater risk, pushes doctors, hospitals, and others into making choices between skimping on actual treatment or closing up shop altogether.

Chapter 3: Why Reimbursement Isn't Reimbursement

There is a scene in Lewis Carroll's *Through the Looking Glass* in which Alice is speaking with Humpty Dumpty. In the course of their conversation, she notices that he uses words to denote things other than their accepted meanings, such as using the word "glory" to mean "a nice knock-down argument." Alice challenges this in the following exchange:

> "But 'glory' doesn't mean 'a nice knock-down argument'," Alice objected.

> "When I use a word," Humpty Dumpty said, in a rather scornful tone, "it means just what I choose it to mean – neither more nor less."

> "The question is," said Alice, "whether you can make words mean so many different things."

> "The question is," said Humpty Dumpty, "which is to be master – that's all."

Humpty Dumpty then goes on to regale Alice with a review of his command of words and their various types and meanings. Alice's experience is a not uncommon experience when dealing with the overlords who make and enforce different aspects of healthcare policy.

One of the first things to understand about the healthcare system is that the bureaucracy is extremely fond of taking words with common meanings and then distorting them to mean something completely different. CMS, its affiliated contractors, and even commercial payers believe they are Master, to use Humpty Dumpty's word, and there is really no further debate or discussion to be had.

"Reimbursement" is probably the most readily accessible word treated in this manner.

We've all been reimbursed for something. Maybe you paid for a friend's meal or offered to fill a colleague's gas tank when they didn't have a means to pay for it. It could be that you went to a training seminar for your employer and had to pay a registration fee to attend. What you (hopefully) received in turn for each of these actions was a like amount of money from each party to make up for the costs you incurred. The very definition of "reimburse" from the Merriam-Webster Dictionary is "to pay back to someone; to make restoration or payment of an equivalent to," with "reimbursement" being the tangible thing that is paid back, restored, etc.

Nobody would ever go out to eat and say that they "reimbursed" the restaurant for their steak. A carpenter or plumber would likely find it extremely strange if the homeowner who hired them told them they would "reimburse" them for their services. In these scenarios, the laboring parties would instead be "paid" or "compensated" for offering a good or service to the consumer. In health care, this is not the case.

Regardless of the payer in question, be it Medicare, Medicaid, or a commercial insurer, those providing services are told they will be "reimbursed" for their work. Accepting this sort of language (and everyone in healthcare does) sets up a couple of perverse relationship dynamics and practical fallacies in how treatment and payment are handled.

First, there is the very basic fact mentioned above that no one fluent in English would use the word "reimbursement" to describe a professional transaction between a skilled worker or facility and those to whom the service or good is provided. Yes, we could use this word for certain internal discussions related to things like expenses an employee might take on for the benefit of an employer, but this is a faulty analogy for the relationship between, say, Medicare and a physician. The physician is not an employee of United Health Care. The physician is not incurring expenses on their behalf. Rather, the physician has a contract to provide certain services to patients (who also have a contract with United) for a certain fee. To call this fee "reimbursement" does substantial violence to the English language and also to the most minimal levels of common sense. Using such an abnormal term creates the impression that the only thing that the health care provider is entitled to is a strictly break-even proposition and that any amount of money above the nominal cost of care is superfluous or unwarranted. Not that this particularly matters, though, given that most Medicare rates don't even reach that level, bringing us to our second point.

The definition of "reimburse," as well as the common understanding of the term, is founded on the cost initially incurred being returned in full. If the training seminar registration cost me $100, then I expect my employer to pay me back the $100. If I fill my colleague's gas tank for $35, his reimbursement to me would be at least that much. Only in healthcare does "reimbursement" entail paying someone back less than the costs of the services they provided. This is a situation seldom known by the average person.

Medicare does not even pay health care providers enough to make up for the cost of seeing Medicare patients. From 2001 to 2014, overall inflation increased by 33.4%. In that same timeframe, physician office expenses increased 60.6% (we'll discuss some of the reasons why later). Concurrent with that period, Medicare payments went up 2.9%.[24] Included in this same era is a 2% pay cut for all Medicare related services that took effect in 2013 and endures to this day as part of budget sequestration.[25] Even CMS's own actuary admitted in 2015 that this trend is unsustainable without causing enormous problems with the Medicare provider base (i.e.- those willing to continue accepting Medicare).[26]

Yet the pressures continue. A survey by the Medical Group Management Association in 2019 reported that 67% of the responding practices received Medicare payments that did not cover the costs of rendering

---

[24] https://www.healthaffairs.org/do/10.1377/hblog20170127.058490/full/

[25] https://www.cms.gov/outreach-and-education/outreach/ffsprovpartprog/downloads/2013-03-08-standalone.pdf

[26] https://www.cms.gov/research-statistics-data-and-systems/research/actuarialstudies/downloads/2015hr2a.pdf

treatment.[27] One respondent lamented that Medicare patients are "more complex, more sickly, [and have] more comorbidities that you don't see elsewhere. It takes more resources to manage their conditions." In other words, a body of patients who frequently consume the most time and resources, therefore generating the largest amount of costs, have their services compensated at an ever-decreasing level, especially when adjusted for inflation.

Some might wonder about hospitals. According to a study by the American Hospital Association in 2016, hospitals were underpaid by Medicare to the tune of $41.6 billion the previous year. That worked out to around 88 cents on the dollar for what was spent taking care of those patients. In a separate report, the ten-year projected effect of Medicare and Medicaid cuts since 2010 totaled $113 billion.[28] Anecdotally, I can say that some of my colleagues have complained of Medicare compensation only covering around 70% of their costs. At least one author suggested that "Medicare For All" proposals would truly highlight this problem in that current Medicare rates pay "only about 65 percent what would

---

[27] https://www.mgma.com/data/data-stories/2019-medicare-reimbursement-rates
[28] https://www.beckershospitalreview.com/finance/aha-hospital-medicare-medicaid-payments-cut-by-113b-since-2010.html

have to be paid for hospitals to have the same net revenue under 'Medicare for all.'"[29]

Again, CMS's own actuary paints a very bleak picture for the future of Medicare rates for hospital inpatient care.[30] Not only that, but the actuary predicts negative Medicare margins for 80% of all hospitals by 2019 and over half experiencing negative total margins by 2040.[31] This latter report manages to be unintentionally humorous by stating, "It should be noted that these simulations are simplistic in that they do not include other factors that could affect margins, such as new efforts by hospitals to improve efficiencies in response to lower Medicare payment updates." In plain talk, this translates to "the hospitals will just have to figure out a way to deal with this."

I have heard some view these numbers as indicating that hospitals are just generally inefficient providers of health care services and should therefore be

---

[29] https://www.racmonitor.com/medicare-for-all-what-about-cost-shifting

[30] https://www.cms.gov/Research-Statistics-Data-and-Systems/Statistics-Trends-and-Reports/ReportsTrustFunds/Downloads/2018TRAlternativeScenario.pdf

[31] https://www.cms.gov/Research-Statistics-Data-and-Systems/Statistics-Trends-and-Reports/ReportsTrustFunds/Downloads/ACAmarginsimulations2018.pdf

forced to streamline their operations if they are to survive on Medicare rates. This imbecilic proposition is countered by data that shows that even efficient hospitals show negative margins when it comes to treating the Medicare population:

> MedPAC saw margins turn negative for relatively efficient hospitals, when the panel assessed 2016 data. The median Medicare margin fell to -1% for efficient hospitals… In this year's report, which assesses 2017 data, the median Medicare margin slipped even further, to -2% for relatively efficient hospitals. These efficient hospitals remained profitable because they had a median non-Medicare margin of 11%, resulting in a total median margin of 8% for 2017.
>
> The median Medicare margin for the other hospitals in MedPAC's sample was significantly worse: -9%. These less-efficient hospitals had a median non-Medicare margin of 9%,

resulting in a total median margin of 5% for 2017.[32]

The cumulative cuts to hospital revenue since 2010 from federal sources will reach somewhere in the neighborhood of $253 billion by 2029.[33] As can be seen in the diagram below, the cuts, enacted by 11 different pieces of legislation, are spread across over half a dozen different areas that dictate how these facilities are paid.

<hr>

[32] https://www.healthleadersmedia.com/finance/medpac-even-efficient-hospitals-cant-cover-costs-medicare-reimbursement. As we shall see later, some of the measures of "efficiency" here include items that are largely out of the hospital's control, such as readmission rates. Hospitals taking care of older, poorer, and sicker patients will naturally be deemed to be more inefficient under this sort of analysis. This further demonstrates that the payment cuts and policy directives we are examining will disproportionately harm the providers and, by extension, the patients who are in most need of help.

[33] https://www.aha.org/system/files/2018-06/estimate-of-fed-payment-reductions-to-hospitals-following-aca-2010-2018-report.pdf

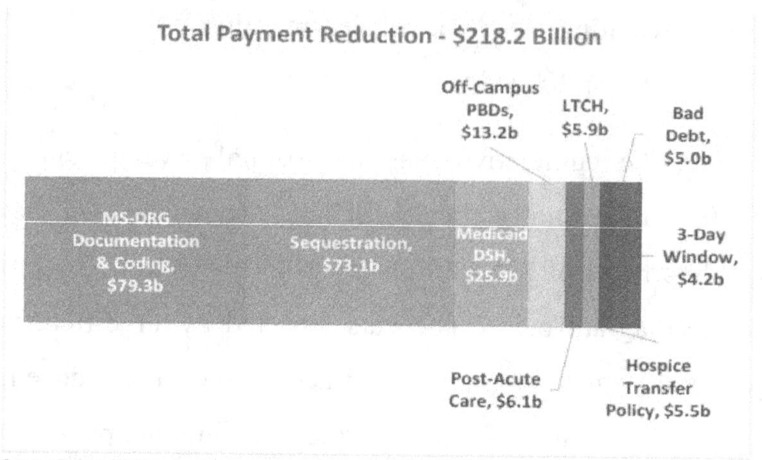

Source: Dobson|DaVanzo estimates – sources and methodology described below.

There is no sign of this phenomenon stopping or even slowing down as politicians look for more and more ways to pay less and less money.

Providers treating Medicaid patients are in much the same dilemma. As we discussed earlier, many Medicaid patients have a difficult time finding a primary care or specialist physician to care for them.[34] This is typically because of Medicaid's lower "reimbursement" rates. According to a 2013 article in Forbes,[35] Medicaid was paying 61% of the Medicare rates for outpatient physician services.[36] Moreover, the same article points

---

[34] A 2013 report from the CDC indicated that 68.9% of physicians were accepting new Medicaid patients: https://www.cdc.gov/nchs/data/databriefs/db195.pdf.

[35] https://www.forbes.com/sites/peterubel/2013/11/07/why-many-physicians-are-reluctant-to-see-medicaid-patients/

[36] As Medicaid programs may vary by state, it is conceded that this

out that "these patients often required much more time and attention than the average patient." This is because, like Medicare patients, Medicaid patients tend to be sicker and have more complex issues than those covered by commercial insurance.[37] This can be for a variety of reasons, but it is a well-accepted axiom for these patient populations:[38]

> Several explanations for inherent differences in payer populations have been suggested. Factors including decreased access to health care, language barriers, level of education, poor nutrition, and compromised health maintenance have all been suggested. However, there is no question that payer status has significant implications on multiple processes of health care delivery.

number may be more or less generous depending upon the practice location.

[37] https://www.beckershospitalreview.com/quality/gallup-medicaid-beneficiaries-sicker-with-chronic-preventable-diseases.html

[38] https://www.ncbi.nlm.nih.gov/pmc/articles/PMC3071622/

Differences exist in not only access but also in the type of primary care that Medicaid and Uninsured populations receive compared with Private Insurance patients…In addition, the Medicaid and Uninsured populations often present with more advanced stages of disease, a reflection of cost prohibitive health maintenance, delayed diagnosis, and the higher incidence of comorbid disease…Other social and lifestyle factors, including drug and alcohol abuse, psychiatric illness, obesity, and high-risk behavior, may further contribute to differences in payer group populations. The impact of the economic burden of poverty may also influence

patients' ability to seek
medical care and to be
discharged from the hospital
in a timely manner due to
lack of support and resources
to be cared for properly at
home.

Hospitals are no different. Medicaid payments had a shortfall of $20 billion compared to costs in 2016. This worked out to be 88 cents on the dollar.[39] Naturally, all of the other complications that make physicians accepting Medicaid more difficult will apply here as well, only more so. A patient sick enough to be admitted to a hospital will typically be sicker than a patient who is in need of an office visit, will typically need more extensive medical intervention, and will, of course, generate a higher cost.

The following graph from the CMS actuary[40] shows the payment levels of Medicare and Medicaid for

---

[39] https://www.aha.org/system/files/2018-01/medicaremedicaidunderpmt%202017.pdf
[40] https://www.cms.gov/Research-Statistics-Data-and-Systems/Statistics-Trends-and-Reports/ReportsTrustFunds/Downloads/2018TRAlternativeScenario.pdf

physicians' practices as a percentage of the payment levels from private insurance.

Figure 2. Illustrative comparison of relative Medicare, Medicaid, and private health insurance prices for physician services under current law

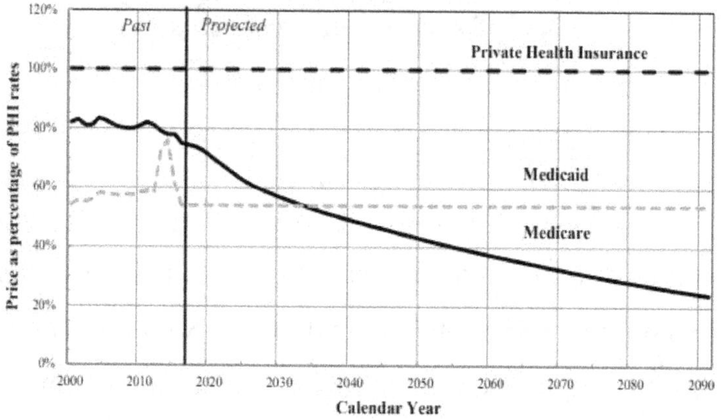

As stated by the actuary report, "Medicare payment levels in 2016 were about 75 percent of private health insurance payment rates, and Medicaid payment rates in 2008 were about 58 percent. In this illustration, Medicaid payment rates increase to 73 percent of private health insurance levels in 2013 and to 77 percent in 2014 before falling to 54 percent for 2016 and beyond."

As stated above, hospitals fare no better.

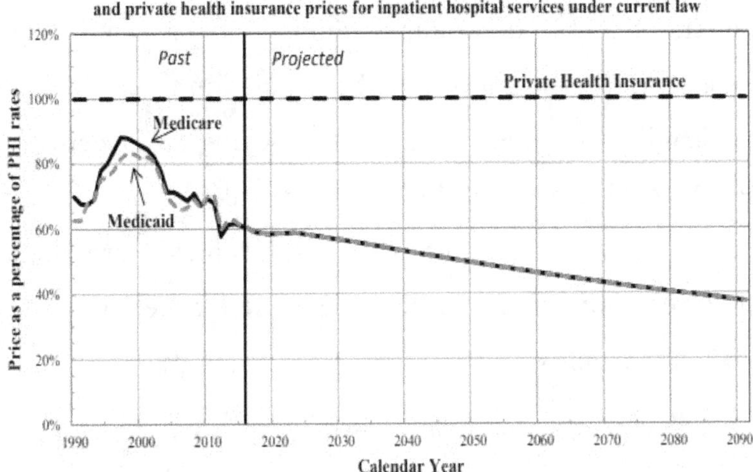

In a similar commentary, the report says, "Medicaid payment rates equal Medicare payment rates in 2016, and both decline in tandem relative to private health insurance payment rates over the next 75 years…By the end of the long-range projection period, Medicare and Medicaid payment rates for inpatient hospital services would both represent roughly 37 percent of the average level for private health insurance."

When faced with more complicated patients for less money, most people would find it completely rational for physicians to limit the number of Medicare and Medicaid patients they see. That is a common practice and regularly taken for granted in the Medicaid space.

The national average for physicians accepting new Medicaid patients hovers around 70%.[41] Quoting this statistic can be misleading, though. In a state like Louisiana, where almost 40% the population is enrolled in Medicaid,[42] only 56.8% of the physicians are accepting new Medicaid patients. In New York, almost one-fourth of the population is covered by the Medicaid program. However, only 57.1% of physicians were accepting new Medicaid patients.

More so than that, a 2014 national investigation discovered that almost half of the physicians who were listed as accepting Medicaid were not available to service the patients, either because they didn't actually accept Medicaid, could not be found at their last known address, or some other reason.[43] Even ones who were treating the Medicaid population often had lengthy wait times, with over one-fourth having wait times of over a month and another one-tenth having wait times of over two months. One pediatrician was quoted as saying, "It's nearly

---

[41] https://www.kff.org/medicaid/issue-brief/data-note-a-large-majority-of-physicians-participate-in-medicaid/; See https://www.cdc.gov/nchs/data/databriefs/db195.pdf for 2013 data from the CDC.

[42] https://www.apnews.com/8439c485a9bb4165b4528939429a704b

[43] https://www.nytimes.com/2014/12/09/us/politics/half-of-doctors-listed-as-serving-medicaid-patients-are-unavailable-investigation-finds.html

impossible to find specialty care for Medicaid patients of any age with diabetes, asthma, sickle cell anemia, and certain other chronic illnesses." This was during a time of rapid Medicaid expansion due to the ACA, so we can only expect the access problems for Medicaid patients to have gotten worse.

Paying no attention to the evidence at hand, CMS has now proposed to eliminate any oversight by states of the link between provider rates and access to care.[44] As the rule stands now, states are mandated to track the existing Medicaid fee schedule rates and determine the effects of those rate levels on patient access. If that scrutiny is taken away, states could then "reduce reimbursement rates to fee-for-service providers without having to demonstrate to the CMS that the rate reductions won't reduce access to care." We will encounter this matter again in the chapter on Medicaid managed care.

What has raised many eye-brows in the last several years is the number of Medicare providers who are following suit. This has been a trend since 2010, the first year CMS had over a hundred physicians opt-out of the Medicare program. "But those numbers jumped to

---

[44] https://www.modernhealthcare.com/payment/repealing-medicaid-access-rule-could-vastly-lower-provider-pay-say-opponents

over 1,600 opt-out requests going into effect in 2013, more than doubling to over 3,500 in 2015, and spiking at 7,400 in 2016."[45] In 2017, an additional 3,732 joined them. As with the Medicaid numbers, this varies from location to location, with Fargo, North Dakota boasting a 100% acceptance rate as compared to New York City's 76%. A study by the Texas Medical Association in 2016 showed only 65% of its members were still taking new Medicare patients. Some will try to paint the decline in opt-outs from 2016-2017 as a sign the trend is reversing, but the deeper picture is more troubling. With the retirement wave of the baby boomer population hitting and over 10,000 new potential Medicare enrollees coming on the market every day, thousands of physicians leaving those patients' access pool every year is a crisis.

There are a plethora of reasons for their doing so, as mentioned by the referenced report. Doctors have shown less and less interest in Medicare participation as the program's reimbursement has not kept up with the cost of providing care and regulations have increased, according to Donna Kinney, director of research and data analysis at the Texas Medical Association. "Between

---

[45] https://www.modernhealthcare.com/article/20180130/NEWS/1801 39995/fewer-doctors-are-opting-out-of-medicare

price controls and the administrative burden, there is real concern about Medicare," Kinney said.

Keep firmly in mind that these are just numbers reflecting the number of physicians opting out of the program entirely. This does not include physicians who are still in the Medicare program but are declining to take on any new patients. The American Academy of Family Physicians claims a membership of 131,400 doctors. Of those, 91% participate in Medicare but only 83% are taking new patients.[46] These are not encouraging statistics for a country looking at 10,000 individuals a day who will be looking for a physician in an environment where almost one in five will be unwilling to take their primary means of paying for their health care.

This is not limited to minor players in the healthcare industry. The CEO of the Mayo Clinic, Dr. John Noseworthy, ignited a firestorm of controversy in 2017 when he announced that his organization would be prioritizing patients with private insurance over those covered by Medicare or Medicaid.[47] This was due to a "surge" in Medicaid patients. That "surge" amounted to a

---

[46] https://www.aafp.org/about/the-aafp/family-medicine-specialty/facts.html
[47] http://www.startribune.com/mayo-to-pick-privately-insured-patients-amid-medicaid-pressures/416185134/

3.7% increase in Medicaid volume, largely due to the ACA expansion. As indicated by Mat Keller of the Minnesota Nurses Association, the fact that private insurance is given priority isn't really a new story. The new story is that "a high level executive actually said it out loud." This was at a time when Medicare/Medicaid patients made up around half of Mayo's volume. After being threatened with a civil rights investigation,[48] Dr. Noseworthy walked back his comments, expressing "regret" over the incident.[49] For what it's worth, Dr. Noseworthy left Mayo Clinic in December of 2018, after also acting as a health care advisor to the Trump administration. He currently serves on the board of directors for UnitedHealth Group as well as Merck.

The numbers here have actually gotten much worse recently. The Medicare Payment Advisory Commission (MedPAC), whose primary role is to advise Congress on healthcare-related issues, especially as it relates to payments, had to cut its calculation of primary care physicians in the US by 20%. Prior calculations had listed almost 46,000 physicians as engaged in primary care when they were actually providing hospitalist

---

[48] https://www.statnews.com/2017/03/17/mayo-ceo-insurance/
[49] http://www.startribune.com/mayo-ceo-regrets-word-choice-about-medicaid-policy/416629323/

(inpatient only) services.[50] While the decrease didn't indicate a problematic lack of access to care at the moment, "MedPAC is concerned by a steep decline in the growth rate of new primary-care physicians, which fell from 0.7% to -0.6% in 2017… It's worried that Medicare beneficiaries might have a harder time gaining access to primary care if the relative number of primary-care physicians goes down long term."

In the end, the entire "reimbursement" system is a very bad joke. Private insurance is obviously not an alternative for these patients because of the high prices of commercial insurance policies. It goes without saying that the older and poorer elements of the population do not contribute large amounts of dollars in terms of taxes.[51] If they are simultaneously creating large expenses through the Medicare and Medicaid programs, the only way to balance the books in this situation is to limit their ability to create those expenses.

The providers who are treating the oldest and poorest (and typically sickest and most infirm) patients are paid less than their costs for doing so. This naturally

---

[50] https://www.modernhealthcare.com/medicare/declining-growth-primary-care-docs-has-medpac-worried-about-access

[51] This is not to say that they contribute nothing nor that they do not contribute large percentages of their income in sales taxes, fees, and other payments to government agencies.

encourages more and more providers to restrict the number of these patients for whom they are willing to provide their services. The older and poorer patients therefore have fewer access points to these services and therefore go untreated, whether for minor illness, such as a cold, or for more chronic conditions, such as diabetes. This will eventually have a positive impact on government budgets in the long term, since these patients will be at a hardship to find a provider who will treat them and then bill the government payer for the service. Viewed from the government's budgetary responsibilities, it will be even more beneficial as these individuals die from their worsening conditions. After all, dead people are incapable of generating new health care expenses.

Of course, one could imagine a scenario wherein healthcare services would be properly funded with additional revenue or the bloated mass of the healthcare regulatory complex (as shall be described later) could be cut to allow for a more streamlined healthcare system. One could even conceive of a project by some politicians to curb the number of services covered by Medicare/Medicaid or other direct cuts to the programs. One can also imagine a society of benevolent alien unicorns coming to Earth and curing all illness and disease with magical gumdrops. The events are all equally realistic.

No additional revenue will be allowed because there is no political will for the taxes to provide said revenue. No real cuts will be made to the regulatory complex because the legislators do not understand the system they are supposedly overseeing and are incapable of knowing what cuts should be made without the bureaucracy's input. The bureaucracy, naturally, will defend itself against any such cuts. No direct cuts to the payer programs will be made because they would set off a media conflagration that would mean a bad outcome in the next election. The government therefore shakes hands with The Reaper and forces providers out of the market, allowing them to absorb any negative backlash and leaving patients without treatment.

If you need a concrete example of how the political spin operates in this realm, look no further than the debates around the ACA or President Trump's recent budget proposal. In the case of the ACA, President Obama and Congress cut over $700 billion out of Medicare in order to fund other parts of the law. The rationale was that "The majority of the cuts...come from reductions in how much Medicare reimburses hospitals and private health insurance companies (Medicare Advantage plans)" [52] and that this was just fine because "the savings…do not cut a single guaranteed Medicare benefit."[53]

I should mention here that "savings" is another oft-abused word in the political lexicon. If you happen to hear a politician talking about the "savings" to be had from a particular healthcare policy, it actually means "cuts."

In the Trump budget proposal, the exact same misdirection is used. In discussing the massive Medicare cuts in the Trump budget, the analysis from the Committee for a Responsible Federal Budget states that "Of those roughly $500 billion in Medicare cuts, about 85 percent of the cuts come from reductions in Medicare's payments to hospitals and doctors, not in cuts to seniors' benefits…"[54] As Avik Roy points out in Forbes:

---

[52]
https://www.washingtonpost.com/news/wonk/wp/2012/08/14/romneys-right-obamacare-cuts-medicare-by-716-billion-heres-how/
[53] Obama campaign spokeswoman Lis Smith as quoted by Forbes at https://www.forbes.com/sites/theapothecary/2012/08/16/fact-checking-the-obama-campaigns-defense-of-its-716-billion-cut-to-medicare/
[54] https://thehill.com/policy/healthcare/medicare/433690-analysis-just-a-tenth-of-trumps-proposed-medicare-cuts-directly

But what happens when you reduce payments to doctors? Doctors stop being willing to see Medicare patients. And if you can't actually get a doctor's appointment, what does it really matter what your insurance plan covers on paper? We already see this happening in the Medicaid program, where sick and injured children can't get appointments to deal with urgent medical conditions, because Medicaid so severely underpays doctors relative to private insurers.[55]

What this means is that Medicare might still be available to cover the cost of certain minor surgeries or a basic visit to the doctor's office. However, if there isn't a surgeon, hospital, or primary care physician available that accepts Medicare as payment, either by choice or because

---

[55] https://www.forbes.com/sites/theapothecary/2012/08/16/fact-checking-the-obama-campaigns-defense-of-its-716-billion-cut-to-medicare/

they have closed their doors, there is no value in its coverage. This is what is happening now. Note also that since government payers tend to focus on the elderly and the poor (and consequently, the sickest) populations, any cuts in these areas automatically hit those populations the hardest. Both political parties play this game with your health care. Neither holds a moral high ground and neither is worthy of your trust on this subject. Remember this the next time your president, congressman, or senator waxes poetic about how they really care for our vulnerable citizens, while their opposition are cold-bloodedly seeking to destroy health care access. The likely truth is that both candidates have already accepted the Compromise, whether they do so out of ignorance, malice, or some misguided sense of pragmatism.

This is, of course, complicated by the fact that CMS tends to act in an utterly lawless fashion with almost no accountability whatsoever. Very recently, a group of over 600 hospitals has been forced to sue CMS for cutting hospital payments for 2018 and 2019 when Congress only gave it authority to implement the reductions for 2014-2017.[56] CMS will naturally try to cling to this money for as long as possible, and there is no guarantee of any kind

---

[56] https://www.modernhealthcare.com/legal/hospitals-sue-hhs-over-840-million-inpatient-payment-cuts

that the courts will actually find in favor of the plaintiffs. Even if the plaintiffs win, forcing a remedy on such a powerful arm of the government may take years.

This ongoing battle for payment is increasingly the case for health care providers. More and more, government and commercial insurance policies create a lingering element of risk for doctors, hospitals, and others who treat medical conditions by wrapping them up in ongoing responsibilities and commitments to both the patient and payer, usually in spheres completely outside of the providers' influence or control. This is done under the labels of "quality" or "value." As with "reimbursement," these words have little do with the concepts of improving the health of a patient or generating a satisfactory outcome for a surgery. They are really just the payers' excuses for further access restrictions by tapping into the patients' side of The Reaper's Compromise.

Chapter 4: Why "Quality" Isn't Quality and "Value" Isn't Valuable

As stated before in our Humpty Dumpty analogy, it's a popular strategy of healthcare policy lingo to dress up extraordinarily awful concepts in positive-sounding language. To the subject of this chapter, what well-meaning person would object to "higher quality" or "greater value" in their healthcare system? This makes it very challenging to combat these concepts in the court of public opinion. Unless one examines the precise function of these terms, it is difficult to understand just how sinister they are.

Every single criticism of the existing health care system revolves around the allegations of "high cost with low quality/low value." There are usually infographics and charts listing the United States and its standing among other first-world countries in terms of these metrics. Inevitably, the US places either in the middle of the pack or at the far negative end of the spectrum. There is typically little analysis offered for the source of the terms or numbers being used. All that is stated is that Americans aren't getting "bang for their health care buck" and that "a system that prioritizes value and quality" should be implemented to replace fee-for-service.

Just an initial reminder that many of those other countries that you see in those charts illustrating the poor standing of American healthcare are using fee-for-service payment systems.

With this in mind, let's consider the word "quality." When a policy wonk talks about "quality," they are almost inevitably referring to a process more so than an outcome.

For example, if you look at "quality measures," they more often than not look like an extensive checklist that the health care provider is required to complete for their patients. One long-running measure from Medicare mandated for years that hospitals offer education to smokers on the potential health hazards of smoking, as well as information on how to quit. Remember that this is for Medicare patients, a group of people typically over 65 years old.[57] As very few people suddenly take up smoking in their 50s or 60s, it's a safe assumption that these people had been smoking for literal decades at this point. Moreover, it's also safe to say that they were very familiar with the dangers of smoking. If they haven't heard it in the mass media campaigns or noticed the

---

[57] This is still a popular measure for some commercial health insurers.

warning labels on every pack of cigarettes they buy, they had certainly been instructed by a primary care physician or mid-level that it's bad for their health. I suppose we could imagine a patient who has never been sick over the course of decades and never seen any health care provider over that time who is also simultaneously illiterate and never consumes any media of any kind, but for the sake of argument, let's say that such an individual would be in a very small minority.

CMS essentially took it for granted that the patient either belonged to this minority or only saw incompetent health care providers who never bothered to educate them on how bad smoking can be.

Now, I ask you to recall Ivy, our medical student from Chapter 2. Ivy was perfectly capable of discussing smoking cessation with any and all patients who walked in the door. Did her conversations do anything to improve the patients' outcomes? Of course not. It did take up time when they could have been discussing more relevant factors or that the doctor could have been seeing another patient. From personal experience, I can tell you that smoking cessation education usually elicits one of the following reactions: (1) the patient is annoyed/angry that this is being brought up at all, making them less focused and attentive on other instructions, orders, and suggestions from the physician or nurse, (2) the patient is amused, which then tends toward the same attitudes as #1, or (3) the patient verbalizes understanding out of courtesy and assures the educator that they have every intention of quitting, now please leave them alone about it.

Once the educational session was done and documented, this patient encounter would show that the "quality" rendered was excellent because the box for "Smoking cessation education" would have been checked. Did anything in this encounter actually result in the patient being healthier? Was there anything that enhanced the patient's well-being? Or was it just a waste of time and resources on a matter that was ultimately of no benefit to the patient at all?

Remember this when you hear lamentations about the waste in healthcare. I can assure you that more waste is generated by these sorts of measures than any deliberate actions by health care providers.

Another item that was implemented and then later removed was the SCIP-CARD-2 measure, which was meant to ensure that patients on beta blockers had been sure to take them prior to their surgery. This measure was eventually removed when it was discovered that it relied upon research that was connected to the deaths of up to 800,000 patients in Europe over a five year period.[58] One would think that our healthcare overlords would have been a bit more diligent in their reviews before imposing such a rule upon potentially every surgeon in the country upon pain of financial penalty.

For a more current example, CMS currently monitors "quality" when it comes to the treatment of sepsis patients. Sepsis is a worthwhile focus of attention. It is involved in over 250,000 deaths a year and is present in 30% to 50% of all hospital admissions that result in a patient's death.[59]

The SEP-1 bundle is a series of events that CMS wants to see occur on any patient who presents to a hospital with sepsis. Such patients must receive the following: blood cultures within three hours, lactate measurements within three hours of presentation and then repeated at six hours, and antibiotics within three hours. The measure is all or nothing. If any one of these steps is omitted, then the hospital may be subject to penalties in

---

[58] https://www.forbes.com/sites/larryhusten/2014/01/15/medicine-or-mass-murder-guideline-based-on-discredited-research-may-have-caused-800000-deaths-in-europe-over-the-last-5-years/
[59] See n. 64, *infra*.

the form of reduced payments because of its lack of "quality" care.

Here is how this plays out in real life. A patient will come to a hospital emergency department and exhibit all the signs and symptoms of being septic. A physician, who is likely already swamped with other emergency situations simultaneously, recognizes the condition, orders tests to verify, and begins dosing the patient with antibiotics to combat the infection. The patient may experience complications, perhaps even coding, but the diligence and skill of the doctor and other ER staff members are a success. The patient's condition resolves, and everyone is grateful for a good outcome.

The problem is that this physician failed the SEP-1 measure. By not ordering the second lactate test, they have, from CMS's perspective, provided poor "quality" care and their hospital must be punished. Since CMS is the entity that gives or withholds the payments, only its perspective matters. No peer review, lawsuit, or other complaint could come to this conclusion. It is entirely the result of a bureaucratically imposed definition that is utterly divorced from the medical decision-making and the patient's well-being.

Consider a different set of circumstances. In the new scenario, the physician recognizes the patient as being septic and follows the SEP-1 requirements flawlessly. This new physician, though, is not nearly as competent as the one in the prior case. He/she can't adapt to the onset of the patient's complication, was overwhelmed by the preexisting comorbid conditions, or some other factor. Our patient here codes and does not recover. They are dead, and let's say that the physician's inability to give proper care contributed to their demise. No sane individual would want to claim that this physician is superior in their quality of care to the one previously discussed. CMS, not known as having a reputation for sanity, will just ask, "Did he comply with SEP-1? It's a simple 'yes' or 'no' question." This is what happens when you take the common meaning of words and then allow them to be re-defined by an organization that is comfortable bartering away the lives of the population.

At least one study illustrates this quite well.[60] Over 800 sepsis cases were analyzed for compliance with SEP-1. Of those, two-thirds failed. While it was true that failure to meet the measure showed some association with

---

[60] https://www.ncbi.nlm.nih.gov/pubmed/30015667

certain negative outcomes for the patient, the link "was no longer significant after adjusting for differences in clinical characteristics and severity of illness…" In addition, 40% of the failures were due to the failure to order the lactate tests within the allotted amount of time. Failure to administer antibiotics in a timely fashion had the strongest link to higher mortality rates yet was only the cause for failure in 15% of the cases reviewed.

What we are left with is that the most dangerous point of failure was only present in 86 of the 570 failures. The failure to timely test lactic acid levels was almost three times more likely to occur but lacks the stronger link to high mortality rates. CMS, though, treats these as though they are completely equivalent factors by applying exactly the same penalty for non-compliance. Of course, the actual patient outcome is not a consideration at all.[61]

The result of all this is an emphasis on process detached from the patient's well-being. A 2017 study on the effects of pay-for-performance measures actually concluded that such programs "may be associated with improved processes of care in ambulatory settings, but

---

[61] The study determined that "SEP-1 may not clearly differentiate between high- and low-quality care, and detailed risk adjustment is necessary to properly interpret associations between SEP-1 compliance and mortality."

consistently *positive associations with improved health outcomes have not been demonstrated in any setting.*"[62]

What makes this situation even more absurd is that the most recent literature on the subject indicates that no amount of improvement in hospital care improves sepsis outcomes by any significant measure. In a study of almost 600 patients across six hospitals over two years, it was determined that "most underlying causes of death were related to severe chronic comorbidities[63] and only 3.7% of sepsis-associated deaths were judged definitely or moderately preventable."[64] The researchers concluded that "Further innovations in the prevention and care of underlying conditions may be necessary before a major reduction in sepsis-associated deaths can be achieved." In other words, sepsis is a terrible problem, but there is very little that hospitals can do about its mortality rate. The ongoing regulatory reaction takes the opposite approach. Hospitals are going to be forced to treat the problem in a

---

[62] https://www.ncbi.nlm.nih.gov/pubmed/28114600

[63] "The most common comorbidities were metastatic or progressive solid cancer (60 [20.0%]), refractory hematologic cancer (16 [5.3%]), severe debilitating dementia (15 [5.0%]), severe debilitating stroke (12 [4.0%]), or severe chronic lung disease (12 [4.0%])"

[64]

https://jamanetwork.com/journals/jamanetworkopen/fullarticle/2724768

certain way, regardless of outcomes, and then be punished for not doing so, again, regardless of outcomes.

One would think that it might be more of a benefit to the patient for hospitals to be given more resources for treating patients with sepsis, especially those with accompanying co-morbidities, rather than worrying about whether or not the proper series of boxes were checked in the midst of trying to save a person's life.

On a different front, recall the Triple Aim that we discussed in Chapter 2. The three axes it used to measure quality were cost, population health outcomes, and patient experience. These are supposedly reflective of "value" in the healthcare system. "Value" is often used loosely as being identical with "quality." This is true to the extent that both words have no real meaning except what is imposed by payers. Something might be a "value/quality" measure today and gone tomorrow at the stroke of a bureaucrat's pen (as was the case with the smoking cessation education mentioned above). For a good exercise in just what "value" means, the University of Utah set up a survey designed to examine what different healthcare stakeholders, ranging from consumers to providers to employers, thought about the concept of "value" and how they would define it. The survey focuses on cost, quality, and service. However you might define those terms is, of course, part of the analysis. Taking the survey between yourself and some colleagues might provide some insight as to just how flexible these terms can be.[65] An article in the Harvard Business Review commented that when patients picked "key characteristics of high-value health care, a plurality (45%) chose 'My Out-of-Pocket Costs Are Affordable,' and only 32% chose 'My Health Improves.' (In fact, on patients' list of key value characteristics, "My Health Improves" was slightly below "Staff Are Friendly and Helpful.") Given the chance to select the five most important value characteristics, 90% of patients chose combinations different from *any* combination chosen by physicians."[66]

Even alleged experts can't agree. Humana recently convened a panel of 18 experts ranging from managed care organizations like Centene to the philanthropic sector such as the Robert Wood Johnson Foundation. The stated purpose was "to build a consensus on the definitions of oft-used but rather nebulous concepts such as 'value-based care' and 'population health.'"[67] The panel couldn't

---

[65] You can find the survey at https://uofuhealth.utah.edu/value/

[66] https://hbr.org/2018/02/we-wont-get-value-based-health-care-until-we-agree-on-what-value-means

[67] https://www.fiercehealthcare.com/payer/humana-convened-experts-to-define-value-based-care-they-failed

reach any consensus of the sort about what either term means. Whether it was debating the presence of patient satisfaction as a "value" metric or trying to determine the best way to group various populations to be measured, the group could not come to an agreement. This, of course, does not stop the government and insurance companies from imposing their arbitrary definitions on physicians, hospitals, and other health care organizations.

In more technical settings, "value" does tend to have a slightly more nuanced meaning. Where "quality" frequently admits that it is focused on process rather than outcomes, "value" almost always purports to be outcomes-based, occasionally with an emphasis on cost as well.[68] In order to increase "value" along these lines, CMS decided that it needed to create the Value-Based Purchasing Program (or VBP) for hospitals.[69] The idea was to pay hospitals based on their performance and how much "value" they provide to their patients. And who can argue with that? Doesn't everyone want to see more value in any transaction that engages them? The VBP sets up a

---

[68] It is sometimes linked to cost with the formula being {value = quality/cost of care}.

[69] https://www.cms.gov/Outreach-and-Education/Medicare-Learning-Network-MLN/MLNProducts/downloads/Hospital_VBPurchasing_Fact_Sheet_ICN907664.pdf

number of metrics for analysis and cuts the reimbursement for the lower performing facilities. The money that is cut is then given to the higher scoring facilities. Those at the median level receive no cuts or additional compensation. With that in mind, let's start our analysis of "value" and the VBP by going directly to one of the foundational concepts of the Triple Aim, namely, patient experience.

Patient experience is just another way of saying "patient satisfaction." The explosion of social media has already put a significant amount of pressure on all health care providers to offer the best patient experience possible. If they don't, they can expect to see negative ratings on Google or commentary from upset patients or patient family members on Facebook or Yelp. Of course, the health care entity has very little recourse to combat this kind of negativity. Suing the patient or patient family member is likely to generate more negative public opinion. Patient privacy laws factor in as well. If the patient's second cousin happens to post on Twitter how incompetent a hospitalist was in caring for their relative, the hospitalist or hospital can't counter by providing medical details showing how the course of action taken was appropriate. This all sets up an atmosphere where providers and facilities must try to be as accommodating as possible in order to avoid criticisms that might drive patients into the arms of the competition. Naturally, this effect is multiplied when direct financial penalties are imposed for having low patient satisfaction scores.

To that end, CMS imposed the Hospital Consumer Assessment of Healthcare Providers and Systems (HCAHPS). HCAHPS is basically a patient satisfaction survey that is sent to a Medicare enrollee after they are discharged from the hospital. The survey questions come directly from CMS. The administering of the survey must be done by the hospital itself, either directly or by hiring a third-party vendor. This, of course, is a new cost to the hospital that it must account for in its budget and, since these are for Medicare patients, the odds are that the hospital has already lost money on providing their care.[70] The first effect of HCAHPS, then, is to increase the cost of taking care of those on Medicare.

When the surveys are returned, CMS uses it to calculate the hospital's VBP score and then cuts those with lower scores. CMS will defend this program by claiming that patients with higher satisfaction scores will be more engaged with their care and more likely to be compliant with the directives of whatever their treatment

---

[70] As discussed in Chapter 3 on Reimbursement.

is after discharge. Having given you the official rationale/excuse/fantasy behind VBP, let's take a look at reality.

Imagine a diabetic patient admitted to the hospital. Any respectable clinician will prescribe this patient a diabetic-compliant diet during their stay in order to help in their recovery. It is a metaphysical certainty that the diet prescribed will not taste as good as the patient's normal, day-to-day fare. Because this patient, like so many others, has signed on to The Compromise, they demand to be provided with "real food," regardless of the effects that it will have on their recovery. Immediately, the hospital is faced with a dilemma. It is certainly in the patient's best interest that they eat the food that is part of their treatment plan. On the other hand, if the patient doesn't get the sort of meal that they want, they will likely bury the hospital on their HCAHPS survey. Most hospitals that I have encountered will take the hit on the survey and serve the patient the compliant meal. Even when they do so, it's fairly typical for the patient to send a family member or friend to the nearest pizza, fried chicken, or other fast food establishment for their "real food." The patient then gets what they want, all the while castigating the hospital for "not caring about them" by trying to force them to settle for bland-tasting food.

An even more common scenario is the chain smoking patient who demands to be allowed to smoke their standard regimen of tobacco, despite being admitted to the hospital for respiratory disease or even for post-operative care. Most hospitals have policies that they are a smoke-free campus. Many facilities, including ours, offer nicotine patches and other similar coping methods to patients who have a smoking habit. That said, I know that our facility regularly has patients sign out AMA (Against Medical Advice) for no other reason than they were told they could not smoke on the premises because (a) it would hinder their recovery and (b) smoking is simply not permitted. I'm sure that any patient satisfaction survey they might fill out would be filled with all sorts of colorful metaphors about the wicked staff who callously offered nothing more than a deaf ear to the patient's desperate need to light up.

On an even more sensitive note, consider now the patient who, for whatever reason, is experiencing or claiming to experience a high level of pain. The physician might offer them Tylenol or some other non-narcotic medication, such as Toradol. Perhaps these work. Perhaps they don't or perhaps the patient in question is drug-seeking. It might even be that the patient is over-dramatizing their pain or that the physician doesn't want to take any chances of hitting a negative survey score for the hospital. The dilemma now is whether to administer narcotics to the patient or risk a bad HCAHPS result. Again, most will risk the survey hit and the resulting impression on the patient that the hospital "just doesn't care."

In the midst of an opioid epidemic, CMS would very much like everyone to forget the initial HCAHPS surveys that had a specific focus on pain management. One question even asked, "During this hospital stay, how often did the hospital staff do everything they could to help you with your pain?" Any patient could always mark a low score here if they didn't receive a narcotic. In 2018, the questions were changed to focus on "communication" about pain, rather than pain management. CMS further demonstrated its part in The Compromise when it removed the responses to the pain questions from affecting the overall VBP score. What they fail to mention is that the final questions on the survey of "Rank your hospital experience from 1-10" and "Would you recommend this hospital" are both absolutely going to be affected by a patient not getting the sort of pain control that they want. Hospitals are therefore still in the same boat. Does a patient get what they need, even to the financial detriment of the facility, or do they get what they want in order to see a bump in the patient satisfaction scores?

These are just a couple of examples, but it's possible some readers are still skeptical about my criticisms. Sadly, the existing literature demonstrates that high patient satisfaction scores actually correlate to higher mortality rates. In other words, the most satisfied patients are the ones most likely to die. The most prominent study came from UC Berkeley several years ago.[71] It has been ignored by policy-makers. The conclusion does not equivocate:

> In a nationally representative sample, we found that higher patient satisfaction was associated with lower emergency department utilization, higher inpatient utilization, greater total health care expenditures, and higher expenditures on prescription drugs. The most satisfied patients also had statistically significantly greater

---

[71]

https://jamanetwork.com/journals/jamainternalmedicine/fullarticle/1108766

mortality risk compared with the least satisfied patients…

Patients typically bring expectations to medical encounters, often making specific requests of physicians, and satisfaction correlates with the extent to which physicians fulfill patient expectations. Patient requests have also been shown to have a powerful influence on physician prescribing behavior, and our findings suggest that patient satisfaction may be particularly strongly linked with prescription drug expenditures…

In a nationally representative sample, higher patient satisfaction was associated with increased inpatient utilization and with increased health care expenditures overall and for prescription drugs. Patients with the highest degree of satisfaction also had significantly greater mortality risk. These associations warrant cautious interpretation and further evaluation, but they suggest that we may not fully understand the factors associated with patient satisfaction. Without additional measures to ensure that care is evidence based and patient centered, an overemphasis on patient satisfaction could have unintended adverse effects on health care utilization, expenditures, and outcomes.

This confirms the real-life scenarios painted above are not some mythical construct of the frustrated hospital's collective imagination.[72] This is what happens with real patients who present with a need to be seen. What's more is that, for all the governmental wailing about the need for "value" and "quality," the policies that drive patient satisfaction scores "had statistically significantly greater mortality risk." People are dying at higher rates, yet these measures and policies endure.

Certain skeptics might ask, "Aren't there objective measures to the VBP system? Those are based on outcomes and aren't tied into a patient's whims, right?

---

[72] See also https://www.beckershospitalreview.com/quality/study-hospitals-with-high-hcahps-scores-may-have-worse-outcomes.html

Those have to increase 'value,' yes?" These are legitimate questions.

Let us then examine some of the more clinically-driven aspects of Medicare's "value-based" engineering of the healthcare system.

The more significant objective outcome-based measures are for the mortality rates for acute myocardial infarction (AMI, essentially a heart attack), heart failure, and pneumonia based on what happens to the patient 30 days after discharge. In other words, if a patient with pneumonia is admitted to the hospital, treated, discharged, and then dies within 30 days, the hospital is penalized for not delivering a high "value" of care. For starters, recall again that these are Medicare patients which, as discussed earlier, means that they will be older citizens and oftentimes sicker than the general population. Recall also one of the fundamental premises of the Compromise, namely, that patients are typically looking for the least bothersome treatment, rather than the most effective one.

First, I should mention that I was unable to find any information that elaborates with specific details on why a 30-day timeframe was selected for these measures, rather than some other number. I can only guess that it was because that number amounts to basically a month.

However, if that is the case, then what is the evidence that indicates that a patient who dies on the twenty-ninth day received less "value" in their treatment than the patient who dies two days later? Perhaps the patient who died on day 29 was a 95-year-old morbidly obese diabetic, whereas the patient who died on day 31 was only 68 and ran three marathons a year. These sorts of questions could go on forever, but the fundamental point is that there does not seem to be any explanation available for why two patients, whether their overall condition is similar or not, could have the "value" of their health care judged simply based on the passing of a few days. If the timeframe selected was only a week, I'm sure the "value" of the treatment rendered would score very highly for most facilities. Likewise, if the measure was based on mortality over five years, I'm sure that scores would reflect almost every hospital performing poorly.

Regardless of the seemingly arbitrary nature of the measure itself, there are other problematic considerations at play in examining post-discharge mortality rates.

Once a patient is discharged from the controlled environment of the hospital back to their home, there is no constraint on their activity or guarantee of health care access. The pneumonia patient may resume smoking three packs a day. The heart failure patient may live in an impoverished area without a readily available pharmacy or clinic. The MI patient may resume their sedentary lifestyle and poor eating habits. One can see how these social determinants of health (as they are now called) could greatly affect a patient's recovery and potential mortality following a serious health episode.

The Kaiser Family Foundation is one of the largest health care analysis organizations in the world. Their data[73] indicates that, generally speaking, the health care a person receives only makes up 10% of the factors relating to that person dying prematurely. The other 90% are items completely beyond the control of any health care provider, with 40% being the result of individual behaviors and 20% as social and environmental factors.[74]

---

[73] https://www.kff.org/disparities-policy/issue-brief/beyond-health-care-the-role-of-social-determinants-in-promoting-health-and-health-equity/

[74] The remaining 30% was attributable to genetics.

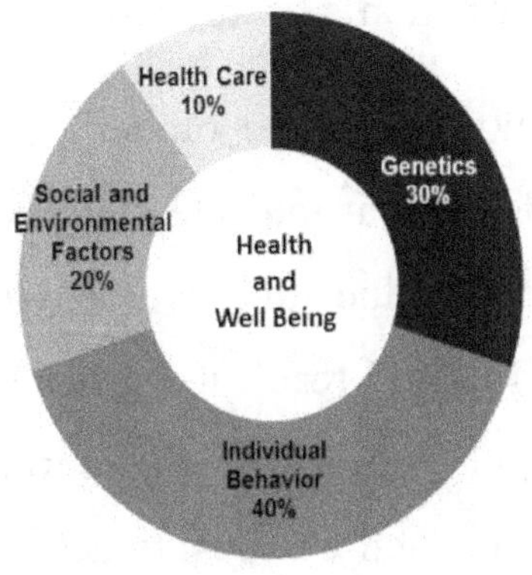

SOURCE: Schroeder, SA. (2007). We Can Do Better — Improving the Health of the American People. *NEJM* 357:1221-8.

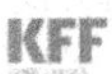

What is in the health care provider's power to restrict any of these life choices or environmental variables? Nothing more than the moral and medical argument that doing these things is bad for the patient's health. Even the book regarded as the bible of health care management admits that there is no way for providers to account successfully for these disparities. "An HCO (health care organization) in a community with high unemployment and low post-high school education should not be directly compared with an HCO in a suburban community filled with professional families…they cannot overcome the social and economic differences."[75] Yet

---

[75] White, Kenneth R. and Griffith, John R. *The Well-Managed Healthcare Organization.* 7th ed., Health Administration Press, 2010.

these comparisons are made all the time and have been codified in the laws and regulations that make up the framework of our nation's health care system.

This is not just some random opinion. There is also ample evidence that indicates the factors confronted by a patient by virtue of their environment and/or personal choices indeed result in higher 30-day mortality rates. One mapped the relevant mortality rates with community factors such as education and income levels. It concluded that:

> Of the social determinants of health (SDOH) analyzed, 79% demonstrated statistical significance within the AMI mortality outcome, 88% in the heart failure mortality outcome and 87.3% in the pneumonia mortality outcome… Due to the disparities in SDOH between urban and rural hospitals, mortality outcomes will shift CMS incentive payments away from hospitals in disadvantaged communities.[76]

---

[76] https://wwww.asc-abstracts.org/abs2019/92-05-hospital-30-day-mortality-rates-are-influenced-by-social-determinants-of-health/

As the risk shift continues from payers to providers, these factors become more and more of a burden on the providers who are the first line of defense. Payers continue to multiply the standards by which they measure the performance of the doctor, the hospital, and so on, yet these standards encompass fields that the provider is unable to affect without significant intrusion into the patient's day-to-day life. Such intrusion, by the way, is something that the vast majority of patients will reject without a second thought.[77]

Another allegedly objective clinical measure that CMS uses to determine as part of its "value-based" health care is hospital readmissions. CMS made its first noises about readmissions as a clinical problem in 2007 following MedPAC's "Promoting Greater Efficiency in Medicare" report to Congress.[78] This report found that readmissions were an unacceptable cost to the healthcare system to the tune of $15 billion per year. While the report conceded that "Not all of these readmissions are

---

[77] One such topic which has seen patient outcry over non-medical questioning and scrutiny of social factors has been physician inquiry into a patient's gun ownership. https://www.washingtonpost.com/news/morning-mix/wp/2016/05/17/have-a-check-up-why-your-doctor-might-ask-you-if-you-own-a-gun/

[78] http://medpac.gov/docs/default-source/reports/Jun07_EntireReport.pdf

avoidable, but some are," it proceeded to recommend public reporting of rates along with financial penalties for facilities that exhibited what were felt to be an excessive number of readmissions. Notice immediately that they concede that it is only "some" readmissions that are avoidable. That ultimately did not stop CMS from punishing hospitals for providing care to the sickest patients among us.

The foundational definition of a readmission for CMS is whether a patient admitted to a hospital for an acute condition is, within 30 days of their discharge, later admitted to another hospital. This counts for any reason whatsoever, excluding only patients who are discharged AMA or whose initial admission was on a psychiatric diagnosis. This means that a patient who was admitted to Hospital A for pneumonia then discharged was delivered low quality care if that same patient, within 30 days of the discharge, fell and broke their hip and had to be admitted for another acute stay (whether at Hospital A or some other Hospital).[79] Under the "value-based" plan to reduce readmissions, any hospital exhibiting an excessive number was to be penalized up to 3% of its Medicare

---

[79] A pdf describing the methodology can be downloaded at https://cmit.cms.gov/CMIT_public/ReportMeasure?measureId=1639 .

payments. The theory was that hospitals would be incentivized to better care during the hospital stay and do more planning and educating during the patient's discharge if it meant money was at stake for not doing so.

Underlying this entire scheme is the idea that any patient who requires a readmission within 30 days must have gotten substandard care or shoddy discharge planning. Is that actually the case, though?

First, there is the problem of determining what actually would constitute a preventable readmission. One project examining all studies of readmissions from 1966 to 2011 noted the extreme variability of the findings in each one and determined the following:

> The proportions of readmissions deemed avoidable varied widely between the studies. This variability makes it difficult to state with any certainty how often readmissions are preventable. Nevertheless, the median proportion of readmissions deemed avoidable (27.1%) is certainly lower than the 76% reported in 2007 by the Medicare Payment Advisory Commission to the US

Congress.[39] Although the variation seen in these studies could reflect true differences in quality of patient care, it also reflects the subjectivity of the outcome itself as well as differences in study characteristics, including patient and hospital types included; factors considered in determining avoidability of readmissions; sources of information used to judge avoidable status; and the minimum number of reviewers per case...

Our study showed that the proportion of hospital readmissions deemed avoidable has yet to be reliably determined. Furthermore, we found a lack of consensus regarding the methods necessary to judge whether readmissions are avoidable. Given the large variation in the proportion of avoidable readmissions between studies using primary data, 'avoidability' cannot accurately be inferred based on diagnostic codes for the index admission and the readmission. Instead, it needs to be determined through a peer-review process in which readmissions are classified as avoidable or not based on expert opinion.[80]

The researchers also noted that, for any readmission reduction project to be viable, it would have to account for multiple factors not necessarily used in the previous studies' formulations. Using the comparison between studies, it concluded that:

> Criteria used in future studies need to focus on determining whether the readmission was preceded by an adverse event (i.e., a bad medical outcome due to medical care rather than the natural history of disease or bad luck); whether the adverse event could have been prevented; and whether the readmission would have occurred even without the adverse event or whether other factors were involved.[81]

---

[80] https://www.ncbi.nlm.nih.gov/pmc/articles/PMC3080556/

These sorts of arguments would seem to be common sense. This, of course, is guaranteed to make them utterly foreign to policy makers at CMS, who instead opted to ignore this list of clarifying factors in order to penalize the greatest number of facilities possible. We see here the same spectre of confusion that clouds all of the other aforementioned attempts to quantify "quality" and "value," namely an inability to say what level of care actually rises to the level of acceptability and why.

Another study[82] further broke down the readmission phenomenon during the 30-day window the readmission occurred. The study looked at over 800 patients in the care of ten different academic medical centers and whether their readmissions showed any distinct characteristics if they occurred in the first week post discharge vs. the readmissions that happened on days 8-30. Of those patients, 36.6% were readmitted in the first week. The remaining 63.4% had their readmission during what was left of the 30-day window.

In other words, far fewer readmissions occur in that first week.

---

[81] *Id.*

[82] https://www.ncbi.nlm.nih.gov/pmc/articles/PMC6247894/

The next measure was to use their own formula for preventability to determine how many of these could have been stopped had there been some sort of medical intervention. Overall, 27.9% of the readmissions were preventable.

Consider for a moment that this also means that over two-thirds of the readmissions were not preventable, a factor that CMS holds in very little regard by treating all the readmissions the same.

Of this 27.9% of preventable (according to this study) readmissions, 36.2% of the early admissions were deemed preventable vs. 23% of the later admissions being preventable. This means that the readmissions that occurred in that 8-30 day timeframe were more likely to have been necessary, rather than something that an additional medical intervention could have mitigated and kept from happening. Again, though, these are treated the same by CMS as the readmissions occurring during days 1-7.

Finally, a qualitative difference in the types of readmissions was detected:

Early readmissions were more likely
to be amenable to interventions
within the hospital, and more likely

to be caused by factors for which the hospital is directly accountable, such as problems with physician decision-making and premature discharge. Late readmissions were more likely to be amenable to interventions outside of the hospital, and were more likely to be caused by factors *for which the hospital has less direct control*, such as appropriate monitoring and managing of patients' symptoms after discharge by the primary care team, and end of life preferences.

In the final analysis then, the study demonstrates that patients who are readmitted within seven days of discharge are those who probably experienced some sort of problem with their actual medical treatment and that these readmissions are more likely to have been preventable.[83] On the other hand, the majority of readmissions come to pass from post-discharge Day Eight onward and are those that occur because of factors that have far less to do with their hospital treatment and far

---

[83] While still admitting that the large majority of readmissions aren't preventable under any circumstances.

more to do with social determinants of health, their primary care follow-up, and so forth.

Why, then, does CMS persist in administering penalties for things that typically happen that are (a) not preventable and (b) only indirectly, at best, linked to the treatment offered by the hospital?

Perhaps the answer can be found in looking at those hospitals most likely to be adversely affected by these penalties.

Several groups have demonstrated that CMS's push for "value" and "quality" are hurting safety-net hospitals, who tend to care for the older, poorer, and therefore sicker populations, with a much greater effect than hospitals catering to healthier, often more affluent patients. One study noted that hospitals in the Mississippi Delta, one of the poorest areas in the entire country, experienced a greater financial hit than peer facilities located outside of the Delta Region.[84]

> "The growing gap in financial performance between the two hospital groups is likely a result of both the amount of penalties incurred

---

[84] https://revcycleintelligence.com/news/pay-for-performance-models-hurt-safety-net-hospital-finances

from HRRP and HVBP, and the expenditure from increased investments in infrastructure for reducing readmissions and improving quality of care and the patient experience," wrote researchers from the University of Arkansas for Medical Sciences, Little Rock.

The analysis of hospital finances between 2008 and 2014 revealed that operating margins were significantly lower at Delta hospitals compared to their peers outside of the 252 counties throughout the period. But the margins significantly fell after Medicare implemented the two pay-for-performance programs…

Total margins followed a similar pattern. Total margins at Delta hospitals dropped from a high of 3.6 percent in 2012 to 0.2 percent in 2014. Conversely, total margins at non-Delta hospitals remained relatively consistent at an average of 5.3 percent…

This is not the only evidence backing up the idea that CMS policy has disproportionately targeted the poor and sick populations for cuts. Another study summarized the mass of data on the subject and came to the same conclusion:

> For instance, hospitals that took care of poor communities were more likely prone to get penalized for hospital readmissions than other hospital organizations…[Residence] in a disadvantaged neighborhood was a hospitalization readmission predictor similar to that of having chronic pulmonary disease… [A] demographic factor categorized as "non-English speaking" was a strong predictor for unfavorable patient satisfaction scores even after taking into account CMS adjustments. The non-English speaking patients were most likely immigrants, who normally relied on safety-net

hospitals and community health organizations for medical care…[Certain] patient panel characteristics (underinsured, minority, and non-English-speaking patients) were associated with variations in physician quality scores. That is, even highly skilled providers still got low scores on pay-for-performance metrics once they took care of greater number of low-income, medically vulnerable patient populations. Similarly, safety-net hospitals and other hospitals that cared for disproportionately higher number of Medicaid patients and black elderly patients were more likely to score worse on quality metrics and penalized. This means that some factors that are not medical in nature like ***"socioeconomic status, health literacy, home environment, adherence to prescribed medications, and the ability to make and keep follow-up appointments"*** do affect quality outcomes measurements and the amount of reimbursements the hospitals are paid for.[85]

The emphasis added above is to highlight the role of the patient's environment and the social determinants of health on the issue. This is widely known among practicing physicians as an enormous piece of the readmission puzzle, yet one that remains well outside of the hospital's reach.[86] In the words of Dr. Greg Marzouka, a Miami cardiologist:

> Unfortunately, the policy ignores patient-related factors that may affect readmissions but are beyond the physician's control. For example, despite my efforts to reduce hospital readmissions for congestive heart failure, I have found that readmission rates plateau because of a small

---

[85] https://journals.sagepub.com/doi/full/10.1177/0951484816678011

[86] At least one study concluded that social determinants of health contributed to over half of all readmissions: https://www.beckershospitalreview.com/population-health/social-determinants-of-health-contributed-to-half-of-hospital-readmissions-study-finds.html

number of patients who are readmitted repeatedly because they are either noncompliant with medical therapy and/or continue to abuse alcohol and illicit drugs. Despite best efforts to set these patients up with home monitoring, frequent cardiology follow-ups, and pharmacy telephone and face-to-face visits for medication counseling, these patients continue to be readmitted 20 to 30 times per year. In resource-poor hospitals, the decreased reimbursement for caring for these patients may inadvertently deplete their already limited funds.[87]

Of course, as we have learned to this point, it wouldn't be a true reflection of The Compromise without showing higher mortality rates for the patients to accompany the financial harm inflicted on the health care providers.

---

[87] https://www.thecardiologyadvisor.com/home/topics/practice-management/are-hospital-readmission-reduction-programs-truly-evidence-based/

It would stand to reason that hospitals faced with crippling financial penalties for readmitting patients would look for whatever ways were available in order to avoid those readmissions. This might be diverting the patient to a lower level of care, sending them home, or perhaps even gaming the system by manipulating diagnosis codes. In fact, at least one study has shown that a "substantial portion" of readmission reductions "are the result of hospital documentation rather than underlying improvements in the delivery of care." [88] Unfortunately, the damage from the penalty program seems to reach much deeper than that.

Recall the research above that indicated that most readmissions are unavoidable and that many have re-hospitalization as the best intervention to deal with the patient's problems. It goes without saying that, when hospitals are forced to administer treatment in ways that are less than what is ideal, bad things will happen to the patient.

A more recent analysis, published in the *Journal of the American Medical Association* in 2018, has indicated that the reductions noted by the readmissions

---

[88] https://jamanetwork.com/journals/jamainternalmedicine/article-abstract/2663252

program correspond with a significant increase in patient mortality. "Among Medicare beneficiaries, the Hospital Readmissions Reduction Program was significantly associated with an increase in 30-day post-discharge mortality after hospitalization for HF and pneumonia…"[89] Moreover, a New York Times article noted that the report came to the same conclusion as the previously mentioned study that any apparent gains were due to "administrative practices, not an improvement in care."[90] It also expressed the real issue, which is whether or not patients might have died because of CMS policy:

> [The research] group have reported, more disturbingly, that the program may contribute to unnecessary deaths. Using the Medicare database to compare mortality rates before and after the penalties were imposed, they found rising mortality within 30 days of discharge for heart failure and pneumonia (but not for heart attacks). The rates of increase were small but growing, and may indicate

[89] https://jamanetwork.com/journals/jama/article-abstract/2719307
[90] https://www.nytimes.com/2019/01/18/health/medicare-hospitals-readmissions.html

that thousands of additional deaths from heart failure and pneumonia followed the program's announcement and implementation.

'Some of those patients previously would have been readmitted, but because of the financial incentives, they were not,' said Dr. Gregg Fonarow, co-chairman of cardiology at the David Geffen School of Medicine at the University of California, Los Angeles, and a critic of the readmissions program.

As one would expect, the Yale University-based team who designed the readmission penalty program denies there is any such danger to patients, saying that this would mean that health care providers were thinking of finances ahead of patient welfare. The hypocrisy involved in this attempted defense is amazing when one considers that the entirety of the readmissions program and the other "value" and "quality" initiatives we have discussed are predicated entirely upon the financial interests of CMS and its desire to lower costs.

Stepping away from the academic ivory tower for a moment to address the issues with those in the trenches, Dr. Fonarow claims that this is absolutely happening, and that they (the physicians) "are getting tremendous pressure from their administrations" over the readmission issue.

While the report eventually waffles on whether or not the program itself is a driver of the higher mortality rate, there is certainly enough evidence linking the program to dead patients to call for restraint. Dr. Steffie Woolhandler at the City University of New York School of Urban Public Health at Hunter College in New York City has expressed similar concerns:

> 'The readmission penalties were always a terrible, terrible idea,' says Steffie Woolhandler, MD, a professor at the City University of New York School of Urban Public Health at Hunter College in New York City.
>
> Unlike MedPAC, Woolhandler believes that only a small share of readmissions is truly preventable. 'Patients with frequent readmissions

are usually very, very sick,' she says. 'We knew from the start that penalizing hospitals on the basis of some percentage of readmissions was not fair and was going to cause problems.'

The program concerned cardiologists in particular, because two of the three initial measures are in that field.

This is a program that had no empirical evidence backing its methodology, no significant pilot testing, and no real idea of what it was targeting to improve. Against all these elements of sound reasoning, it was still imposed on thousands of hospitals in a one-size-fits-all manner. Now, it appears as though people may be dying, and the response is a press release showing "concern." Even today, there are many who argue that the perceived benefits of the readmission penalty are either illusory or "modest at best."[91] One would think that CMS would at least consider suspending the program to allow for a deeper dive into the existing data. Of course, that has not

---

91

https://www.medpagetoday.com/hospitalbasedmedicine/generalhospitalpractice/79145

happened, nor will it, because CMS has to uphold its part of The Compromise.

Basically, this amounts to, "Yes, people are dying, but CMS is saving $2 billion a year. One must have priorities."[92]

This is not even the only example of hospitals being forced into bad decisions due to adverse financial incentives. Starting in 2008 and then increasingly so with the passage of the ACA, hospitals have been subjected to penalties for patient falls. This created an incentive for hospitals to limit patient mobility to the greatest degree practical, even though limiting patient ambulation can be an obstacle to patient recovery from illness or surgery. Whether it's investing in bed alarms to indicate when a patient gets out of bed, excessive use of bed rails, or diverting staff to monitor a patient's movement, hospitals

---

[92] Recently, there has been a well-publicized and much-ballyhooed change in the readmission penalty, ostensibly to mitigate the damage of the penalty for safety net hospitals. This was accomplished by altering the penalty formula by accounting for the number of dual eligibles (those qualifying for Medicare and Medicaid) in a hospital's patient mix. While this is being touted as some sort of revolutionary boon to health care providers, the reality is that the effects of the new formula are minimal. "As a result of the changes, the study estimates that average penalties for teaching hospitals will drop from $287,268 to $283,461... For rural hospitals, their average penalties are estimated to decline from $55,268 to $53,633." https://www.modernhealthcare.com/payment/teaching-rural-hospitals-gain-cms-readmission-changes

have been mandated to limit the falls in the Medicare population and have done so with all the urgency that the financial penalties dictate.[93] Consequently, falls may have been reduced, but it has been at the expense of better overall patient care for the elderly.[94]

The most recent effort to inject "quality" and "value" into the healthcare system has been the imposition of the Medicare Access and CHIP Reauthorization Act (MACRA) in 2015. This legislation was passed with overwhelming bipartisan support, clearing the House of Representatives by a 392-37 margin and passing the Senate by a vote of 92-8. MACRA fundamentally altered the way physicians are reimbursed for their services to Medicare patients by subjecting them to penalties for not abiding by a multilateral data reporting system. The payment system envisioned by MACRA places physicians[95] into one of two categories.

---

[93] https://www.washingtonpost.com/health/overzealous-in-preventing-falls-hospitals-are-producing-an-epidemic-of-immobility-in-elderly-patients/2019/10/11/d1894374-d8ab-11e9-a688-303693fb4b0b_story.html

[94] *Id.*

[95] Please note that, while I use the term "physicians" to describe the parties affected by MACRA, this is merely for convenience purposes. The actual regulations affect nurse practitioners, physician assistants, physical therapists, social workers, and almost every other provider of health care services to the Medicare population.

The first is the Alternative Payment Model (APM). A physician participating in an APM will be providing services under some sort of arrangement that is not fee-for-service. In other words, a physician who is accepting fully capitated or bundled payments for his Medicare population will probably fall into this category. Physicians in an APM will be those with the resources to accept higher levels of risk for their patients' behavior. More than likely, this will mean physicians caring for patients who are relatively healthy and financially well-off and hence carry less inherent risk than poorer, unhealthy patients.

The second MACRA track is the Merit-based Incentive Payment System (MIPS). MIPS is a vast data reporting scheme that is broken down into four separate categories. The first is "Quality," defined by CMS as "the quality of the care you deliver, based on performance measures created by CMS, as well as medical professional and stakeholder groups."[96] Six different quality measures must be reported for the provider or group in question. All are practice specific, so for example, an internist will not be submitting the same data here as, say, a gynecologist. There are hundreds of

---

[96] https://qpp.cms.gov/mips/overview

possible measures ranging from "Tobacco Cessation Education for Adolescents" to "Unplanned Reoperation within the 30-Day Postoperative Period." These measures started out as 45% of the physician's total MIPS score but will decline to 35% by 2021.

The second MIPS category for reporting is "Promoting Interoperability." This metric is structured around the physician's use of an electronic medical record (EMR). While we will discuss the proliferation of EMRs in a later chapter, for MIPS purposes, this basically means reaching a certain level of "sharing test results, visit summaries, and therapeutic plans with the patient and other facilities to coordinate care"[97] and the like that meets governmental satisfaction. This component is 25% of the total MIPS score.

The third MIPS category is "Improvement Activities." This category purports to measure "how you improve your care processes, enhance patient engagement in care, and increase access to care."[98] There are almost 100 different activities to choose from. Physicians must choose up to four different activities, each of those having high or medium point ratings. The physician can carry a

---

[97] *Id.*
[98] *Id.*

maximum of 40 improvement points. Once the four activities and their corresponding point levels are selected and calculated, the number of points achieved in this category is then converted to a number reflecting 15% of the final MIPS score. The activities themselves range from "Provide 24/7 access to eligible clinicians or groups who have real-time access to medical records" to "Participation in a 60-day+ effort to support domestic or international humanitarian needs" to "Use group visits for common chronic conditions."

The final category is "Cost." This was not considered in the initial MIPS scoring but rises to 30% of the total score by 2022 as the other scoring measures decline in weight. The good news for physicians is that they don't have to report on costs at all. The cost numbers are derived entirely from Medicare claims data and automatically factored into the formula. The bad news is that the cost of care for a given patient is the factor most outside of a physician's control (due to the reliance of effective treatments often being the result of patient compliance), as well as being the factor most likely to result in care rationing by the physician. Does the physician admit a patient for inpatient rehabilitation services, which are far more costly, albeit more effective, than outpatient rehabilitation? Or does the physician, cognizant of the cost metric for MIPS, try to send the patient to the less expensive care environment in hopes that it will be equally effective?[99]

This is the dilemma of The Compromise on well-meaning providers. By their reporting year of 2022, MIPS will be cutting physicians up to 9% of their Medicare Part B reimbursement for failing to meet these reporting and practice standards. A physician might have happy patients and deliver good outcomes, but the fact that they choose to care for a patient population with low incomes and high health care needs could very well result in that physician seeing a reimbursement decrease.

Not only is there a reimbursement cut associated with this program, but there is also a significant cost hardwired into the reporting mechanisms. The reporting and submission of this data requires that a health care provider invest in an electronic medical record. These are not cheap, and we will discuss them in more detail in a later chapter. However, for the time being, consider the case of Dr. Barbara L. McAneny, president of the American Medical Association. Dr. McAneny, in an

---

[99] For the truly masochistic, the final 2,379 page rule affecting the Physician Fee Schedule incorporating the MACRA provisions can be read at https://s3.amazonaws.com/public-inspection.federalregister.gov/2018-24170.pdf

effort to be an example to the other physicians of the AMA, went all-in on MIPS and wound up scoring a perfect 100 points. This generated an additional payment to her oncology practice of $34,000. In looking at the net result, though, she found that it had cost her over $100,000 to get that high score.[100]

She is not the only clinician finding that MIPS is "simply not worth it."[101] Another expert comments:

> For all the work involved in reporting for MIPS, many physicians and practice managers across the country are coming to recognize that the 1.68% bonus given from the government's payment program may not be worth the time and resources required to participate… In a typical practice, Medicare Part B reimbursement hovers around $50,000…The bonus, therefore, is at best $840, paid in pennies and dimes throughout the year. And, if history repeats itself, that figure will drop

---

[100] https://www.medscape.com/viewarticle/912790
[101] https://www.medscape.com/viewarticle/916056_1

before any payout is made. Last year, the promise of a 2.05% bonus was whittled down to 1.88% after the government had processed all appeals…

But despite all the downsides and all the costs, it's critical that you participate in the program! That's because the penalties are significant. While there are hopes of gaining $840, there are realities of losing more than 7% in 2021 (the impact year for the current performance year of 2019, as the program runs in 2-year cycles). You can't afford that.[102]

Not only are the payments for participating miniscule, but CMS has a hard time just paying them. As of September 2019, over 90,000 clinicians were still waiting for their APM bonus payments from the data submitted for 2017.[103] There isn't even a reason given for why the payments are delayed. What does this mean for the providers who invested so heavily in the resources to

---

[102] *Id.*

[103] https://www.modernhealthcare.com/payment/providers-still-waiting-2017-advanced-apm-bonuses

participate in the program? It means, of course, that they will eat those costs for as long as CMS holds their money.

The formulas for these payments and penalties are mathematical and fairly fixed. Any policy-maker who really cared to understand the MACRA scheme could have looked at the financial metrics associated with Dr. McAneny's (or any of the above example practices) and told you that this was going to be the result. The truth is that many of them were told how burdensome and financially harmful the program would be. Why, then, did it pass so handily?

The first possible response is that Congress and the President didn't understand the law they were passing. This is possible but fairly improbable. As mentioned above, they were warned. Even if they missed these warnings, someone wrote this law and its enabling legislation, perhaps banking on the ignorance and laziness of our elected officials, similar to the way Mr. Gruber described the ACA as relying on the stupidity of American citizens. Did the Grubers of the world who drafted this legislation somehow not understand what they were writing and its effects?

Highly unlikely.

The second possibility is that those same individuals promoting MACRA knew absolutely what the effects would be and thought those effects were a positive thing. Why would these things be positive? Because they have the long term effect of limiting patient access to care, specifically and especially among the higher cost populations, leading to a decline in claims and money saved.

Regardless, whether it's from laziness or neglect or outright intention, the provisions of The Compromise are manifested quite well by MACRA and its consequences. While common sense demonstrates that more restrictions on how health care can be provided will eventually lead to lower utilization and costs due to patient inaccessibility and mortality, is there any evidence that the focus on "quality" and "value" have an effect?

There is a significant amount of evidence that says that it does not.

In one study, 32 primary care practices were engaged in an initiative to receive a National Committee for Quality Assurance certification and accompanying investments in patient screening and testing for a variety of ailments over a three-year period. While there were large increases in getting boxes checked (such as designing registries to track patients with chronic diseases), there was "statistically significantly greater performance improvement, relative to comparison practices, on 1 of 11 investigated quality measures: nephropathy screening in diabetes." In three years, there was improvement on one out of 11 measures. Not only that, but the main thrust of the entire "quality" push was called into question as participation in the program "was not associated with statistically significant changes in utilization or costs of care."[104]

In summary, what hath the emphasis on so-called "value" and "quality" wrought?

First, it has triggered a vast wave of confusion in the healthcare industry, as nobody can agree on what these terms actually mean.

Second, it has promoted a focus on often superfluous processes rather than whether or not the patient saw improvement in their outcomes.

Third, it has furthered the shift of risk to providers for activities that they have almost no control over whatsoever. In a world of patients prioritizing treatment convenience and lifestyle wants over behavior changes

---

[104] https://jamanetwork.com/journals/jama/fullarticle/1832540

and necessary, but annoying, courses of action, burdening physicians and other health care professionals with these items is absurd. As one colleague pointed out to me, there is a documented link between long-term mortality rates and having a poor sense of smell.[105] Are providers possibly going to be held responsible in the future for their patients' poor olfaction? I probably should not have even mentioned it since it's now likely that CMS will somehow embed smell tests in the next round of "quality" measures.

Fourth, the measures themselves are oftentimes ineffectual and lacking in any firm evidence, as study after study shows that they do not even have the stated goal of increasing "quality" or "value" (if we use those terms to reflect the outcome of the patient's health improving). Even more problematic is when these measures appear to be actually increasing patient mortality, of which there is significant evidence in the case of the patient satisfaction scores and readmission penalties. Despite the correlation, if not causation, associated with these measures and dying patients, CMS continues to plow ahead without any real regard for the consequences.

---

[105] https://www.medscape.com/viewarticle/912322

Fifth, it is indisputable that the enormous task of recording and reporting all the data associated with keeping up with the morass of "quality/value" programs is increasing the cost of healthcare and eating into the margins of physicians, hospitals, and other providers. In many cases, these margins were already negative. This will eventually drive providers out of the market of caring for the classes of patients who need access to care the most.

Sixth, the addition of a MACRA penalty for physicians who try to help their patients by referring them to effective but high cost treatments and settings guarantees that physicians will face an increasing amount of pressure to prescribe patients cheaper, though less effective treatment, in order to avoid being financially crippled for daring to believe that a higher cost alternative would be better for their patient.

I apologize for the length of this chapter. It is an extremely convoluted part of our system and difficult to describe if you are not living in it every day. However, I ask that you imagine yourself in such a scenario. Imagine trying to take care of dozens, hundreds, or even thousands of sick people every day of your life and not being able to focus on the person in front of you and their problems because you are wading through an endless parade of mandates, directives, and other imposed obligations that not only have nothing to do with patient care, but also might have the effect of harming those who have come to you for help. Failure to comply is better for the patients, but it can also mean the potential ruin of your practice or service.

How does one function in such an environment, especially when tasked with saving the life and preserving the health of their fellow man?

Chapter 5: Why Codes Can't Be Decoded

If you've ever utilized the services of a health care provider, you've probably heard the words "code" or "coding" mentioned, especially if there was some sort of problem with the bill you received for the services rendered. To those who are not coders (and even some who are), medical coding is a bit of a mystery that defies a summary explanation. In practice, coding is a highly complex and gravely critical matter. There are dire consequences for using incorrect codes. A health care provider with an incompetent or renegade coder could find themselves facing lost revenue, recouped payments for revenue already received, or even fines and jail time. Ultimately, bills that are generated for health care products or services are tied to a code (or multiple codes) of one form or another. The ability to bill a given payer for that product or service is dependent on the correct code being used.

So what are these "codes" that play such a prominent role in our healthcare system? Just providing a definition is not an easy matter, but we will attempt to give the basics here.

The American Academy of Professional Coders defines **medical coding** itself as "the transformation of healthcare diagnosis, procedures, medical services and equipment into universal medical alphanumeric codes."[106] In essence, it means that different aspects of the health care delivery system are assigned specific combinations of letters and numbers that allow payers to understand what service or treatment was rendered for a certain diagnosis and what the payment will be for whatever the provider did. There are multiple different types of codes, each with its own role in this process.

The **ICD** (International Classification of Diseases) code is the letter/number combination used to identify what a patient's diagnosis is. We are currently on the tenth version of the ICD system, so you will frequently hear these called ICD-10 codes. There are other countries working off the ICD-11 series, but that hasn't been adopted in the United States yet. Certain payers (specific workers' compensation carriers, for example) still use the ICD-9. To give you an idea of the complexity of ICD coding, it's instructive to look at how drastic the change was to go from the ninth series to the tenth.

---

[106] https://www.aapc.com/aboutus/

ICD-9 codes were typically three to five characters. ICD-10 codes range from three to seven. There were around 13,000 ICD-9 codes. The ICD-10 switch contained over 68,000 codes. There were also certain ICD codes associated with procedures, usually those provided on an inpatient. The ICD-9 variety ranged from three to four numbers long in a total set of about 3,000 codes. The ICD-10 contains seven alpha-numeric characters in a total set of over 87,000 codes.[107]

If this sounds like it is excessive, there is a reason for that. The level of detail and specificity required to properly code an ICD-10 claim can approach the absurd. For example, here are some distinct ICD-10 codes for your reading pleasure (yes, these are all real):

1. **Y92.253 – Injured at an Opera House**
2. **W22.02 – Walked into lamppost**
3. **W220.2XD: Walked into lamppost, subsequent encounter[108]**
4. **W61.43 – Pecked by a turkey**
5. **Z63.1 – Problems in relationship with in-laws**
6. **V97.33 – Sucked into jet engine**

---

[107] https://www.ama-assn.org/sites/ama-assn.org/files/corp/media-browser/premium/washington/icd10-icd9-differences-fact-sheet_0.pdf

[108] The patient walked into a lamppost and apparently ricocheted off, only to walk into yet another lamppost.

7. **V97.33XD: Sucked into jet engine, subsequent encounter**[109]

8. **X52 – Prolonged stay in a weightless environment**[110]

9. **V91.07 – Burn due to water skis on fire**

10. **V95.43 – Spacecraft collision injuring occupant**

11. **T63.012A - Toxic effect of rattlesnake venom, intentional self-harm**[111]

I can assure you that there are many, many more that could have made this list.

CPT (Current Procedural Terminology) codes are codes that deal exclusively with procedures or services rendered. Typically done in an outpatient fashion, they are made up of five characters, which may be numbers or letters. There are also three different categories of CPT codes, with the first category being further subdivided into six separate sections. There are now almost 10,000 CPT codes.

The **HCPCS** (Healthcare Common Procedure Coding System) codes are mostly identical with the CPT

---

[109] Yes, this means that the patient was sucked into a jet engine, survived, and then was sucked into another jet engine.

[110] To further establish the lunacy of this particular code, understand that the code series of X51-58 are all designated as "accidental." This means that that patient in question somehow wound up accidentally confined to a prolonged stay in outer space or perhaps a diving tank.

[111] We can only assume this means an attempted suicide by snake.

codes, except for those specifically designated as HCPCS Level II. These are designed to capture services that are not offered in a standard doctor's office or hospital setting. For example, provision of an oxygen tank or a prosthesis would have a HCPCS code, as would an ambulance trip. This sounds simple, but understand that there are at least 16 different sorts of HCPCS Level II codes (A codes, J codes, Q codes, etc.). There are also Level III HCPCS codes that are assigned by state Medicaid programs for certain specific needs their plans might have. Indeed, there are still more varieties we could look at (APCs, NDCs, MS-DRGs, CDTs, and still more), but that would be a book unto itself. This being the case, please accept the above as the most common examples and not as an exhaustive list.

It's very easy to mock this system. Whether it's the absurdity of the ICD-10 codes mentioned above or just the thought that billing for anything at all in health care takes place against this kind of backdrop, there is plenty to make fun of. However, any laughter on the subject quickly fades away when a provider is confronted with the enormous burden that coding diligence requires.

The health care billing process usually works by a service being rendered. That service is connected with one or more of the aforementioned codes. The code is connected to a charge. The code and charge are then applied to a claim form, which is then transmitted to a payer for payment. If the ICD-10 code is incorrect, whether by being completely wrong or just not specific enough, the payer may deny the claim due to a lack of medical necessity. If the CPT or HCPCS code is entered for a lower charging procedure or patient encounter, the payer may send money, but it will only be a fraction of what was merited by what was actually done for the patient.

In other scenarios, the consequences may be even worse. A provider may innocently be mistaken on what the proper code for a given instance might be. Given the thousands upon thousands of coding variations, this is quite common. However, in this case, the provider might be coding for something that garners more payment, rather than less. The payer will then seek to recoup its monies from the provider, leading the provider to engage in costly appeals and other protective action. Perhaps the provider will be accused of medical billing fraud or abuse, leading to fines or even jail time.

A 2014 HHS study reviewing 2010 claims data determined that $6.7 billion was paid inappropriately for that year. "That amounted to 21% of Medicare payments and a staggering 42% of incorrectly coded claims. In fact, the $6.7 billion that was inappropriately paid disguises the extent of the problem, due to the fact that the incorrect coding included both upcoding and downcoding, with the *majority* of incorrect claims being downcoded."[112] The picture is of a large number of claims getting paid at too high of a rate, while a vast host of other claims aren't being paid enough. This could be either out of a lack of competency among the coders, or, given what I've seen in my personal experiences, an extremely conservative posture by practices to make sure that they are not subjected to audits, recouped payments, or any of the other penalties that may be levied for upcoding.

On a more subtle level, coding results in problems that are a bit more abstract from what we see in the day-to-day delivery of health care. By way of example, when a payer looks to adjust for the risk posed by a given patient, it will often do so by extracting the coding data for that patient and determining how sick that patient is based on whatever diagnoses and treatments have been coded. This risk adjustment will allow the payer to project how expensive this patient might be for it to hold as a

---

[112] https://www.m-scribe.com/blog/bid/353427/improper-e-m-coding-leads-to-loss-of-revenue-for-practices

client. Patients demonstrating very high risk scores will see higher increases in their insurance premiums.

Government contracted plans, like those in the Medicare Advantage program, can receive more payments from CMS if they can show that their patients are sicker than the average Medicare recipient, promising billions in additional revenue for documenting as many ICD-10 codes on each patient as possible.[113]

The complications spawned by the coding system go even beyond that, though. Recall all the worthless and nonsensical "quality" and "value" measures that were mentioned earlier. All of these are equally tied to the use of a given code in a given situation. The entire metric can be altered with a simple change of diagnostic coding. One such example is avoiding the pneumonia mortality measure by coding those patients as septic or as suffering from acute respiratory failure. A relevant study determined that 28% of pneumonia patients admitted to a sample of over 300,000 admissions could have been legitimately re-coded with an alternative diagnosis. The study found a "substantial" opportunity for these hospitals

---

113

https://www.modernhealthcare.com/article/20180901/NEWS/1808 39977/insurers-profit-from-medicare-advantage-s-incentive-to-add-coding-that-boosts-reimbursement to improve their scoring in the pneumonia measure by "gaming" the measure that CMS had in place in this manner.[114]

The gaming aspect is not limited to providers. As we've seen, CMS is always looking for ways to cut a provider's payment without actually calling it a "cut." One of the many ways in which it accomplishes this is by manipulating provider codes. The most prominent example of this is scheduled to occur in 2021 when a particular subset of Category I CPT codes, known as Evaluation and Management (E&M) codes, will be changed to accommodate CMS's desire to pay providers less. The standard E&M coding scale was five levels, with each level corresponding to a higher level of intensity for an encounter with a physician. Naturally, the higher, more labor-intensive codes were paid at higher levels than the lower codes. In 2021, CMS will be collapsing the Level 2-4 codes into a single code, and establishing a single "blended" rate, almost guaranteed to be less than what is currently paid for Levels 3 and 4. While this is being done in the name of administrative simplification, it has largely escaped attention that CMS is proposing a variety of "add-on codes" to these

---

[114] https://www.ncbi.nlm.nih.gov/pmc/articles/PMC4617210/

encounters, meaning that, while some meager additional payments will possibly be on the table, there is far more likelihood of additional coding burdens to deal with as well.[115]

We do have some data that provides some help in quantifying exactly how much of a burden this is. A 2018 study[116] attempted to ascertain exactly how much the billing process (including coding) cost providers trying to get paid. This study was performed at a large academic health care system in North Carolina that had consolidated all of its billing activities into a single entity. It also had fully adopted a certified electronic health record in 2014. The results of the study indicated that "the estimated costs of billing and insurance-related activities ranged from $20 for a primary care visit to $215 for an inpatient surgical procedure." This is a telling statistic since a primary care physician is probably only getting around $70-$80 from a Medicare visit for that patient.[117] A commercially insured patient encounter might yield a higher payment but will almost certainly be more costly, a

---

[115] https://revcycleintelligence.com/news/cms-delays-collapsing-of-e-m-payment-rates-until-2021

[116] https://jamanetwork.com/journals/jama/fullarticle/2673148

[117] This is based off of the Medicare payment for a 99213, the E&M code associated with a moderate-intensity patient follow-up visit to a primary care physician lasting around 15 minutes.

fact mentioned in passing by the study. Generally speaking, Medicaid payments for the same visit will be much lower yet will involve much more in the way of resources to claim payment due to the proliferation of managed care systems in the Medicaid environment.[118] In other words, for a basic primary care encounter, a physician could be paying up to one fourth of their Medicare payment just for the privilege of being able to bill Medicare at all.

The point illustrated here is to demonstrate further that there is an enormous amount of costs in our healthcare system that have nothing to do with patient care. In all the political rambling shoved down our collective throats about the costs of health care, you almost never hear a reference to the extraordinary administrative costs. You hear about prices and end-of-life care and the FFS system and greedy doctors/hospitals and so on. Very, very few bother to mention the costs that are nothing more than requirements set by payers as conditions for payment. The New York Times reported[119]:

---

[118] The impact of managed care on the Medicaid patient and provider populations will be discussed in more detail in Chapter 8.
[119] https://www.nytimes.com/2018/07/16/upshot/costs-health-care-us.html

That New England Journal of Medicine study is still the only one on administrative costs that encompasses the entire health system. Many other more recent studies examine important portions of it, however. The story remains the same: Like the overall cost of the U.S. health system, its administrative cost alone is No. 1 in the world…At just over 25 percent of total spending on hospital care (or 1.4 percent of total United States economic output), American hospital administrative costs exceed those of all the other places…[120] Hospitals are not the only source of high administrative spending in the United States. Physician practices also devote a large proportion of revenue to administration. By one estimate, for every 10 physicians providing care,

---

[120] The survey also examined Canada, England, Scotland, Wales, France, Germany and the Netherlands.

almost seven additional people are engaged in billing-related activities…

Another study in Health Affairs surveyed physicians and physician practice administrators about billing tasks. It found that doctors spend about three hours per week dealing with billing-related matters. For each doctor, a further 19 hours per week are spent by medical support workers. And 36 hours per week of administrators' time is consumed in this way. Added together, this time costs an additional $68,000 per year per physician (in 2006). Because these are administrative costs, that's above and beyond the cost associated with direct provision of medical care…

Costs related to billing appear to be growing. A literature review by Elsa Pearson, a policy analyst with the Boston University School of Public Health, found that in 2009 they accounted for about 14 percent of total health expenditures. By 2012, the figure was closer to 17 percent.

Now, there are a couple of other items to take away from the article. First, there is a slight segue at the conclusion to discuss the amount of cost associated with claiming money directly from patients in the form of copays and deductibles. While these are factors, one must recall that the vast majority of these efforts are focused on the payers. It is implicit in the practice of medicine that some patients are not going to be able to pay their bills. Patients are people with far fewer resources than United or Blue Cross or Medicare. Like any rational actor, the provider is going to pursue payment from the deeper pocket with far more diligence because it is taken for granted that the payer has the resources to pay. That being said, while there are costs associated with patient payments, they are dwarfed by the processes and expense that go toward (a) generating a claim to be paid in the first place, as partially described in this chapter about coding and (b) forcing the payers to pay the claim once it has been submitted.

Second, the article has a small section devoted to describing the administrative cost problem as being associated with the lack of a single payer system in the United States. This is hardly a closed case, as it is clear from the studies cited that the administrative costs in countries with single payers varies wildly from nation to nation. Moreover, it is a base assumption that a single payer system in the United States would result in less administrative burden. While I'm not discounting the possibility, it is foolish to think that the burden would be eliminated rather than simply shifted and consolidated into one entity. The popularity of "quality/value"-based payments and of managed care in the Medicare and Medicaid systems has demonstrated that administrative burden is easily encouraged by public agencies and government contractors.

How does this affect the Compromise? It all harkens back to Mr. Gruber's comments in our introduction. It benefits policy-makers and the payers they are aligned with to make the system as complex as possible, even if the actual treatments and care being delivered are not necessarily so. The more complicated the system is, the more avenues there are for denying claims, withholding payments, or seeking recoupments of monies already paid. The more a provider is forced to add cost in an effort to meet the challenges of this ever-more complex system, the less able that provider is to provide care. The oldest, sickest, and poorest patients are the first ones the provider will shed in order to streamline their operations to get the most revenue out of each encounter. They simply cannot afford to provide these patients care under such a regime.

From the patients' perspective, the more complex the system is, the less the patient will understand the source of their problems. It is fairly commonplace for a patient to call us (or any other provider) to complain about their bill. As much as we might try to explain the ins-and-outs of their payer's reasons for denial, it all typically comes back to the fact that the patient simply does not understand what has happened. Nor really should they. To use the coding example again, the typical coder usually has at least an associate degree and a professional certification for their profession and usually will make between $40,000-$50,000 a year. The average patient, regardless of their education level, is somehow expected to be able to match this in order to unravel the intricacies of their medical bill.

When the time comes to complain, the patient will then tend to direct their anger toward the provider. The nameless and faceless payers, especially in the Medicare and Medicaid spaces, will get off without a single shred of accountability.

I will leave the billions of dollars a year spent on consulting services, outsourcing, and other exact mechanisms for coping with this complexity for another time. Suffice to say, these costs should not be regarded as strictly in-house expenses. There is an ever-growing crowd of "experts" specializing in these areas who are more than happy to help providers deal with the problems. For a fee, of course. Naturally, this expert class is promoted heavily for their views on how to make the system better. Oddly enough, despite being invited to speak at national healthcare conferences, policy think-tanks, government round tables, and the like in order to share their wisdom, I have yet to hear any of them actually propose a sensible solution. And why should they? Steps that actually reduce the complexity of the system would put them out of business.

Having gone through a few of the items that make up the monster that is the health care/administrative complex, I leave you, the reader, with the following diagram.[121] This was produced based on feedback from

[121] https://www.cms.gov/About-CMS/Story-Page/Complexity-and-Burden-of-Hospital-Reporting.pdf

the staff and leadership of health care providers in an attempt to graphically portray the administrative burdens associated with the industry. We have talked about some of these. Others are in the coming chapters. Still others are so complicated that it would take volumes to describe them in detail (e.g.- cost reporting and its associated appeals).

When looking at this, try to establish what links these activities might have with taking care of sick people. Also, recall that most of the design was, in all likelihood, produced by people who do not engage in taking care of sick people and therefore have no concept of what it entails. Finally, remember that those who did design it were in actuality seeking ways to (a) avoid payments and (b) kill provider access to older, poorer, and sicker populations in order to keep costs lower.

Complexity and Burden of Hospital Reporting

Between May and June 2018, 151 hospital staff and leadership shared their experiences with reporting information to external and regulatory entities. This graphic illustrates the reporting interactions that pull hospitals away from their central focus of patient care and the burden they experience.

REPORTING INTERACTIONS

A - Caring for Patients

Providing patients with coordinated healthcare

A1 Sending patient health records, medical orders, and prescriptions to other providers, facilities, and suppliers

B - Accreditation and Certification

Establishing and maintaining compliance with patient health and safety requirements

B1 Submitting corrective action plans for citations captured on Form CMS-2567 following an accreditation survey

B2 Submitting corrective action plans for citations

B3 Responding to complaint surveys conducted by the state on behalf of CMS

C - Quality Reporting

Abstracting, submitting, and improving performance on quality measures

C1 Submitting core measures, Electronic Clinical Quality Measures (eCQMs), and hospital-acquired infection data

C2 Submitting quality measures as required by Accrediting Organization

C3 Submitting quality measures as required by the state

C4 Submitting quality measures as required by other payers

D - Utilization and Case Management

Reviewing utilization of benefits and managing patient care across providers

D1 Reviewing CMS coverage rules and guidance

D2 Coordinating care with other providers and exchanging patient health records

D3 Reviewing other payers' coverage and coordinating benefits

E - Cost Reporting

Gathering financial data, filing annual cost report, and settling accounts payable to or receivable from Medicare

E1 Submitting cost report and filing cost report appeal

F - Coding, Billing, and Appeals

Coding patient records, billing payers, and appealing denied claims for reimbursement

F1 Submitting claims, appeal letters, and documentation to MAC

F2 Submitting claims, appeal letters, and documentation to other payers

G - Individual Provider Enrollment

Credentialing, verifying, and enrolling providers to bill to Medicare and Medicaid

G1 Submitting credentials and application for state licensure

G2 Submitting Medicaid provider enrollment application

G3 Submitting provider enrollment application to commercial payers

G4 Submitting Medicare provider enrollment application

BURDEN EXPERIENCED

Varying Standards

Hospitals must balance varying requirements from multiple regulators. Interpreting and reconciling overlapping rules takes excessive time, resources, and brainpower. Hospitals wish their regulators could all get on the same page and write consistent standards.

Areas where this burden is felt most:

A B C D F G

Duplicative Reporting

Hospitals provide the same information to a number of entities in slightly different formats. This redundancy increases the complexity of reporting and associated costs. Due to its mostly clinical nature, duplicative reporting pulls clinicians off the floor into reporting tasks and roles.

Areas where this burden is felt most:

A B C D F G

Pace of Change

Hospitals are constantly reacting to new CMS rules. They develop new Electronic Health Record (EHR) modules, revise policies, and retrain staff. They want to slow down, plan proactively, and develop sustainable systems. At the same time, they expect standards to stay current with evidence-based care.

Areas where this burden is felt most:

A B C D F

Insufficient Dialogue

When hospitals seek to clarify CMS requirements, they often receive responses that cite the requirements—or hear nothing back at all. When hospitals want CMS to change something for the better, they feel like no one listens. Hospitals feel ignored and wish for more dialogue with CMS.

Areas where this burden is felt most:

A B C D E F G

Lack of Transparency

Despite the volumes of requirements imposed by CMS, hospitals feel that CMS operates in an inscrutable "black box." They wish they had more visibility into CMS oversight methodologies and logic behind the requirements.

Areas where this burden is felt most:

A B C D E F

Chapter 6: Why Charges Aren't Prices

There is a particular delusion that is currently sweeping the country as it pertains to prices in healthcare. Whether it's from the White House, pundits, or policy-makers, there is a widespread belief that the problem of health care delivery and costs can be remedied by the silver bullet of more transparency in what providers charge for their services. The idea is typically stated in terms that confuse the healthcare marketplace with the marketplace for other goods and services in the economy.

With other items, prices make for a sensitive measure as to the desirability of a good/service to a consumer. The consumer has to determine if the price in question is what they want to pay. If a cheaper option is available, they will usually buy the cheaper option, barring any concerns about quality or more amorphous factors like personal brand loyalty. This effect of prices is well-known, so competing suppliers of the good/service have an incentive to keep their prices as low as possible. If their prices ever outstrip those of the other competitors, they run the risk of losing customers to the other supplier.

If this works in so many other fields of commerce, why is healthcare different?

As mentioned in the previous chapter, when a diagnosis and treatment for a patient are coded, that code is associated with a particular charge for the service. That charge is then used as a basis for the compensation the provider receives from the payer. However, it is not accurately described as the "price," at least, not if we regard the price to be what is actually paid for the service in question.

Think of it in terms of visiting your local car dealership. If you are shopping for a car, you will be presented with a lot full of numerous models, each one bearing a sticker with an amount of money that you can pay to own the car. Anyone could pay that money and walk home with a vehicle. However, nobody ever pays the sticker price. There is a negotiation. The charge listed on the sticker goes down. Modifications might be made to the vehicle sale itself (additional features, extended warranties, etc.). Still, the patron acquires ownership of the vehicle and pays an actual price far different from what was displayed.

So it is with healthcare.

Hospitals keep an entire list of their charges for every single service code they provide. This list is called a chargemaster. Recent federal action required that every hospital in the country publish their chargemasters on the hospital website. This has been done. Yes, there are cases where the data in question is formatted in a difficult manner, but the charges and corresponding codes are there. What is consistent among them all is that they all change when they are submitted to a payer.

Let us begin with Medicare. Medicare essentially pays based on a fee schedule. In other words, CMS and its contractors have a list of what they actually pay for any given code submitted. If the fee schedule says that the provider is to be compensated up to $100 for a given code then that is all Medicare pays. The patient may also be responsible for deductibles, copays, or coinsurance associated with the coded service, but these are not set by the provider. They are determined by Medicare. The provider could also charge less than the Medicare fee schedule: say, $90. In that case, Medicare would pay the charged amount.

On the other hand, the provider in question is certainly free to charge as high a rate as they want for the service. They might charge $100 or $1,000,000. It is irrelevant. The payment from Medicare will be the same. The deductibles, copays, and coinsurance will be the same, hence the patient's out-of-pocket expenses will be the same. The provider writes off the difference between the payment made and the charge listed as an "explicit price allowance."[122]

Under these circumstances, the charges are irrelevant as long as they rise to the level of the Medicare fee schedule. Again, a provider could choose to charge less than the Medicare rate, but since we know Medicare is usually paying less than the cost of the service anyway, why would the provider choose to take less? With the patient's out-of-pocket cost being beyond the provider's control, any incentive for the provider to lower their charges is effectively eliminated. The charge will rise at least to the level of the Medicare fee schedule and go no lower. The patient remains unaffected regardless of the charges. Whether at the $100 charge or the $1,000,000 charge, every patient in this scenario will be on the same playing field in terms of what they have to pay.

Now, consider the Medicaid patient. Like Medicare, Medicaid also typically pays according to a fee schedule. The charge cannot compel a payment of more than what the Medicaid fee schedule allows. As a program for lower-income individuals, Medicaid also, with rare exceptions in certain states, prohibits any sort of

---

[122] Formerly known as a "contractual allowance."

collection directly from the patient. There are therefore no copays, deductibles, or coinsurance amounts left over from a Medicaid encounter. As before, the provider may charge Medicaid whatever they choose. Charging more will not yield a higher payment, though, so the remainder is written off.

As with the Medicare patient, the charges involved mean nothing. Assuming the provider acts in a rational fashion and sets their charges at least equal to the Medicaid fee schedule, Medicaid will pay the one amount. The patient will pay nothing, regardless of the charge level. Again, there is no incentive whatsoever for the provider to lower their charge out of some sort of concern that the patient will go elsewhere for their care due to a competitor being cheaper.

On a side note, recall that Medicare rates are commonly much higher than Medicaid rates. Providers are prohibited from setting different charges to patients depending on what sort of insurance coverage they have. This means that the provider will have one charge for each service code. That being the case, if a provider has set their charges at the Medicare fee schedule level, they will almost certainly be in excess of what the Medicaid fee schedule would be.

Let us now move on to the patient carrying commercial insurance. Contracts between commercial insurance carriers and hospitals, doctors, etc. can provide for payment terms in a variety of ways. Until the last decade or so, it was fairly common to see commercial insurers pay claims based on a percentage of the provider's charge. In other words, Blue Cross would agree to pay Hospital X 50% of whatever the hospital's charge for a given service code was. This naturally created an incentive for charges to be increased over time. Eventually the insurers reacted against this trend and restructured their agreements for providers in their network.

Now, it is far more common to see payer contracts that compensate the provider based on either a fee schedule, similar to Medicare and Medicaid, or by what is known as "referenced-based pricing," which basically operates by taking a percentage of whatever the Medicare fee schedule allows.

In the former case, the fee schedule will pay the provider at a much higher rate than the Medicare fee schedule and therefore be much more lucrative to the provider. The provider, in turn, agrees to accept the insurer's auditing and review terms, their network conditions, prior authorization standards, and so forth. In turn, the provider agrees to accept less than its charges, whether this is by direct discounts or by adhering to the payer's fee schedule. The basic exchange here is that the provider agrees to be part of the payer's network, gaining access to the payer's covered patients, in exchange for giving discounts to the payer for claims that are filed. Now, part of this entire arrangement also includes the collection of deductibles, copays, and coinsurance from patients.

As a reminder, let's recall what these terms mean. The **deductible** is an amount of money that the insured patient agrees to pay before the insurance carrier agrees to begin paying claims at all. If a patient has an insurance policy with, say, Anthem, that has a $1,000 deductible, then the patient will have to pay $1,000 out of pocket before Anthem begins picking up payments for any part of that patient's claims.

Copays are specific, fixed amounts of money that patients are required to pay upon receiving health care services. These amounts, while fixed, may vary based on the service being received. A patient may have to pay a $20 copay any time they go for a primary care visit. A visit to a specialist's office, though, might require a copay of $40. Imaging, such as a CT or MRI, might mean a higher copay than that, and so on.

Coinsurance is the amount of money a patient is left to pay after their insurance kicks in once the deductible is met. Once a patient has paid the $1,000 deductible mentioned above, they might require a hospital stay. Let's say that the hospital is in the payer's network and has a contract with the insurance company to accept a fee schedule rate of $5,000 for the entire time the patient is admitted. The charges might be $10,000, but yet again, this is irrelevant because the hospital has agreed to accept the $5,000 as compensation. The patient's insurance policy states that the patient is required to pay a coinsurance of 20%. The patient then pays 20% of the compensation to the provider, while the payer pays the remaining 80%.

Notice that, even in this case, the charges are meaningless. A patient, knowing the charges in advance, would be able to decipher what their out-of-pocket costs would be. Those costs are not so much a function of the charges, though, as they are a function of the contract their insurer has with their insurance company, coupled with the terms of their own insurance policy. The patient could have perfect knowledge of the charges of every single hospital in a 100-mile radius. The charges for these hospitals might vary from the $10,000 in our example to $25,000 at another hypothetical facility. However, if the terms of the payer's contracts with the facilities still call for the same basic fee schedule, the patient's responsibility at the end of the day has not changed one cent. Now, I readily concede that the contracts might vary a great deal, but this will likely not be affected by what the facility is charging and will depend more on things like the facility's market share, the negotiating strength of the insurance carrier, and other such related items.

We can perhaps come up with scenarios wherein charges might have some sort of meaning. If a patient has no coverage at all, they will be billed for the full charges of whatever sort of encounter occurred. Remember the analogy to the sticker price of an automobile, though. A patient billed $10,000 for an inpatient stay, who has no assets or significant income, and is very likely unable to pay, will be in a strong position to negotiate a significant discount from the provider. The provider knows good and well that there is only so much blood one can get from a stone and that something is better than nothing. It will negotiate with the patient for a much reduced rate. The discount will be steep, and the patient, while still perhaps being faced with a daunting bill for someone of their means, will not be compelled to pay anything close to $10,000.[123] In this particular case, the charges do have some meaning because they will serve as the baseline starting point for any of this negotiation. Still, the provider will have to face the same reality of the patient who is unable to pay and will therefore still seek a similar, albeit perhaps not entirely equal, discounted rate.

This sort of situation might also present itself in the case of a patient seeing an out-of-network provider. One would expect these situations to be limited to emergencies or encounters where the patient is unable to determine if a provider is in-network or not.[124] Here, the patient's insurance policy will shift more, possibly even all, of the responsibility for the provider's compensation onto the patient. Eventually, this results in a similar situation to the uninsured patient. Let's say the insurance policy requires the patient to pay 100% of the charges for any out-of-network provider. If that's the case, they will receive the "sticker price" bill and will then be in a

---

[123] In 2016, talk show host John Oliver was famously able to discharge $15 million in medical debt for a mere $60,000.

[124] For example, a situation in which a patient undergoes surgery at a particular in-network hospital with an in-network surgeon. Unbeknownst to the patient, the anesthesiologist is not in network, and the patient's insurance therefore refuses to compensate him/her for this service as it does the in-network providers, leaving the patient with a larger portion of the bill, possibly up to 100% of the billed charges.

position to negotiate it downward from there. The provider will again be forced to offer a discount for some payment, rather than potentially receive nothing or far less than the discount if the patient is forced into bankruptcy or destitution.

I do understand that patients with very high deductibles, network difficulties, or no insurance coverage at all might benefit from knowing the charges in advance. If a patient was confronted with a $5,000 deductible but needed something expensive like an MRI, for example, they can shop around for the lowest charge provider, negotiate a cash price based on those charges, and pay the cash price without being confronted with the full cost of their deductible or the pressure of negotiating the reduced rate after the bill for the full charges has come to their doorstep. However, when reflecting upon the limiting number of factors for this to be effective (a premeditated encounter, a specific coverage situation calling for a need to negotiate, etc.), it is extremely difficult to see how this resource-intensive push for price transparency is supposed to create some sort of seismic shift in how patients and providers interact.

With all of these factors in play, there is little to no incentive for providers to reduce their charges. Even the aforementioned federal mandate that all facilities publish their charges on their websites is fairly meaningless. Is the potential ability to squeeze additional money from an uninsured patient with little means (the only party for whom charges hold any meaning) on an already discounted number worth dropping charges below the Medicare or commercially contracted rate? Of course not. Yet policy wonks would have you believe that this publication of pricing will immediately allow patients to shop among hospitals, forcing them to compete for the business of those uninsured patients, resulting in an overall decrease in charges across the board. Having reviewed the entire process in this chapter, I hope readers can discern why this prediction is a pipe dream.

One can see how additional transparency might even lead to further chaos in the system. As of this writing, the Trump administration has proposed an additional rule for hospitals that would also require them to post their negotiated rates with commercial insurers. This would allow public access to the fee schedules that United, Blue Cross, Aetna, and so forth pay for "at least 300 'shoppable services' consumers might consider beforehand, such as X-rays or lab tests."[125] This sounds

---

[125] https://www.cnbc.com/2019/07/29/trump-proposes-hospitals-publish-prices-negotiated-with-insurers.html

all well and good. A hospital might charge $3,000 (to use round numbers) for an MRI, but United's fee schedule might be 33% less than that charge. Remember, providers give insurance companies these discounted rates in order to be granted in-network status with the insurer, thus guaranteeing the provider a supply of patient volume from that insurer's members. United, therefore, pays $2,000 for the MRI, and the hospital can feel comfortable knowing that patients with United insurance will utilize its facility for services.

A patient without insurance or perhaps with a $5,000 deductible would be in a position to call the hospital, knowing that United only pays $2,000, and offer the hospital that amount for the MRI. The hospital will happily take the $2,000 and provide the patient with the treatment. However, is the patient's lot all that improved? They could have offered $2,000 (or far less) and likely had their offer accepted by the hospital regardless of their knowledge of the pricing structure for United. Does this help the patient knowing that United pays $2,000 at one hospital vs. $1,500 at another vs. $3,000 at another? Probably not as much as is being projected, as any of those hospitals would have accepted a cash payment at a deeper discount than what they discount the insurer in the first place. Recall that the hospital has already paid for the

MRI machine and the salary of the rad tech performing the scan. It isn't going to be subjected to any large additional costs for conducting this patient's additional scan.

The result, then, is that the patient has a starting point for a negotiation but not much more. As is the case with shopping in the car lot, the patients fitting into this subset of the larger population still only have a sticker price that is largely irrelevant to what they will actually pay for the service.

Is there a potential downside to all of this transparency on insurer discounts? Yes, and it is a considerable one. If everyone knows what discounts a provider is negotiating with an insurer, the negotiations largely become worthless. For example, a provider might negotiate with Aetna to accept a fee schedule that averages out to be a 25% discount off of its charges in order to be in Aetna's network. At the same time, they are working on a contract with United for the same services. United might be a bigger priority for the provider, so they would be willing to take a fee schedule that averages out to be 33% less than the billed charges. If the latter discount rate has to be published, Aetna will immediately know that United is being offered a better deal. They, in turn, will demand the same discount being offered to United. Every provider in the country will find themselves in this scenario and with a significant chunk of negotiating leverage stripped away.

On the other hand, insurers will essentially be given a license to collude with each other and to set compensation for providers at a specific rate for them all, regardless of what the provider's business model or existing margin happens to be. Again, when Medicare and Medicaid don't cover the cost of taking care of a patient, providers are forced to make up that loss with what they are paid by commercial insurance. With so much of their bargaining power with insurance companies gone, providers will inevitably see their margins shrink or go negative.[126]

All of this raises the question of why charges are at their current levels in the first place. After all, we've all heard the stories about how a Band-Aid or a Tylenol in a hospital setting is marked up to some apparently obnoxious degree. As with the other scenarios, this is

---

[126] I concede there may be certain markets where a hospital or physician group could hold such a monopoly on a given service that they would always have an insurance company over a barrel. However, at this time, this is likely an extreme minority. The continued acceleration of provider mergers may eventually change this balance of power.

often an indirect factor of providing health care services. In this instance, it relates to the language used by every single payer in existence for their terms of reimbursement.

Whether it's Medicare, Medicaid, or some commercial payer, each one agrees to pay according to its fee schedule/reference based price or billed charges, whichever happens to be *less*. This means that if the provider's charges are less than what is otherwise guaranteed by the payer, then they will get that lesser amount only. What does this motivate the provider to do? Raise their charges, of course.

As we've already seen, Medicare and Medicaid typically do not even cover the cost of the care rendered. What provider would therefore want to get paid even less? Charges are therefore, at a minimum, set at the Medicare level.[127] What about those commercial payers, though? Since Medicare and Medicaid pay less than cost, that loss has to be made up somewhere. The provider will therefore set their charges at a sufficiently high level so as not to find themselves leaving money on the table because

---

[127] Keeping in mind that Medicare almost(?) always pays more than Medicaid.

they charged less than what their payer contract would allow.

Nor are providers in a position to simply set their charges equal to or just on the cusp of what commercial plans will pay. Each commercial contract will likely pay different rates. With that being the case, the provider charges will at least be equal to the highest rates their most lucrative commercial payer is willing to pay. Otherwise, again, that provider leaves money on the table that would be better put to use making up for their Medicare and Medicaid losses.

Another question that might be asked is why there are not different charges for different payers. There are two considerations that prohibit this as a resolution, one practical and the other legal.

From a practical standpoint, this would enormously increase the complexity of the revenue cycle process. Maintaining and updating a single list of charges for each and every one of the thousands of codes mentioned in the prior chapter is already difficult. Multiplying that list by the number of payers a provider might encounter would likewise multiply the amount of personnel and resources dedicated to that task.

From the legal side of things, there are very strict rules about not discriminating against patients based on their payer. If a provider was to begin charging for its services based on whether the payer is Medicare vs. commercially insured, there could be potential risk of these sorts of claims arising and the fines and sanctions that go along with them.

Regardless of the above measures taken, the following remain guaranteed:

1. Charges will never fall below Medicare fee schedule rates.
2. Charges will never fall below the lowest commercial insurance fee schedule rates.
3. Because of ongoing renewals of commercial insurance contracts, providers will continue to raise their charges to stay ahead of fee schedule changes.
4. No amount of transparency will change any of these items for patients.
5. Current proposed transparency rules will allow for collusive rate setting for insurance companies, boosting their margins and hurting provider compensation rates, with patients likely getting no benefits whatsoever.

In summation, this massive focus on charges by crowds of talking heads, media personalities, and politicians is essentially worthless. The charge reflects a number that nobody pays. The only events that occur that even result in a consideration of charges are subsets of subsets of the thousands of patient encounters that occur in a day, and those are oftentimes driven by adverse patient choices (e.g. seeking care with out-of-network physicians or hospitals). Charges certainly don't reflect the cost of care, nor do they have any bearing on the impending insolvency of our government payers since those payers dictate their payment levels to the provider.

You don't have to take my word for it. Consider the words of Merrill Goozner, editor of Modern Healthcare magazine:

> Among all the proffered panaceas for reducing America's high healthcare costs, price transparency is the least likely to make a major dent in the problem...Price transparency is largely irrelevant for Medicare patients, since the CMS pays the same to every provider, adjusted for local

conditions. State Medicaid agencies also pay common rates and set strict limits in how much their impoverished clientele will pay out-of-pocket…While [charges] matters a lot to the 30 million people who are uninsured, their rack rate bills usually get written off as charitable or uncompensated care…While [commercial based plans] looks like a textbook case for price transparency, there's not much incentive for any of these patients to switch to a lower-priced provider. Their out-of-pocket expenses won't change since each will pay the same deductible at each hospital. The cost of the operation everywhere is well above their out-of-pocket limits, even in the high-deductible plan. This helps explain why only 10% of prospective patients use price comparison tools when they are available.[128]

The focus on charges does make for a convenient tool to distract from the actual problems with the healthcare system, though. Venting our collective societal spleen against "greedy doctors/hospitals" allows for a toxic injection of emotion into the headlines and encourages the thought that "something should be done!" Sadly, anything done here will provide nothing more than wasted time and kudos to policy-makers for their continuing accomplishment of nothing all that helpful.

128
https://www.modernhealthcare.com/article/20190216/NEWS/1902
19967/editorial-the-transparency-trap
It should be noted that Mr. Goozner claims to be in favor of greater price and quality transparency because it will "expose institutions that are outliers" in those categories. However, he gives no indication of how that might happen or how relevant any such information might actually be.

Chapter 7: Why Payers Aren't Payers

Much of the previous information has been provided in order to lay the foundation for a very basic, yet often overlooked, premise. It is another example of common language not accurately reflecting reality. We often refer to Medicare, Medicaid, United, Aetna, Blue Cross, etc. as "payers." The truth is that they only perform the function of "paying" when they are absolutely forced to do so. The main purpose of their existence is actually quite the opposite. Their main purpose is to conceive of (a) ways not to pay or (b) ways to recoup monies they already paid.

As has been shown above, there is an endless, ever-changing, and always innovating series of obstacles placed between the health care provider and the compensation for their services. Even in the event that the compensation is rendered in a timely manner, there is absolutely no guarantee that they will be able to keep it. Whether it takes the form of absurd penalties for matters beyond their control, direct cuts to a fee schedule, or audits and recoupments years after the services were rendered, not one penny of a provider's money remains safe.

I submit that there is not a single industry in the world that lives with such uncertainty to its cash flow.

While this is ultimately true of any so-called "payer," each sort goes about it in a different way, so we will examine them in turn. Each of these will lay bare the goal of half of The Compromise participants, so the significance of grasping this cannot be understated.

Let's begin with traditional Medicare and a metaphor to illustrate just one method CMS uses to target providers.

Imagine the scenario of a restaurant. A patron (we'll call him Joe) visits the restaurant in order to obtain its services in preparing and serving food. The restaurant provides Joe with a steak and shrimp dinner, and he willingly pays for the meal with a gift card. Joe leaves satisfied, while the restaurant staff move on to serve the next customers who arrive. Joe himself may be long-forgotten, but the record of his meal purchase is maintained by the restaurant owner.

Two and a half years later, a third party appears, claiming to be acting in the interest of Joe and the gift card company. They accuse the restaurant of having accepted too much money for the meal that was served.

Moreover, they claim that Joe should have received an entirely different meal based on what was paid. The third party then demands that the entire amount of the meal be returned to the gift card company, minus a small commission for themselves as the collector. Then, the third party, without actually reviewing other meals or bills, simply declares that the restaurant must have engaged in similar behavior with more of its patrons and requires the restaurant pay back the monies for 25% of all the meals that were purchased with a gift card like Joe's. The restaurant, of course, can challenge this through the proper legal channels but, while it waits years for its case to be heard, the third party gets to keep the recouped money.

This entire scenario sounds ridiculous and absurd, yet it describes the procedures taken by Recovery Audit Contractors (RACs) on a regular basis all across the country. RACs were initially created by the Medicare Modernization Act of 2003 as a demonstration project and then later expanded by the Tax Relief and Healthcare Act of 2006. They are private companies engaged by CMS to audit fee-for-service Medicare claims, usually for proper coding or medical necessity. The RAC is paid on a contingency basis, meaning that they are incentivized to find problems and demand money back from the provider, whether the provider actually did something wrong or not. Ostensibly, this is done to prevent providers from committing some sort of fraud and getting paid by Medicare for something they didn't do. As we shall see, this is merely more jiggery pokery window dressing from the government meant to conceal its own malicious behavior.

The parallels with Joe's meal at the restaurant would go something like this. A patient goes to a hospital that treats chronic wounds. During that patient's encounter, an excisional debridement of the patient's wound occurs.[129] The physician (who let's say for simplicity's sake is employed by the hospital) performing the debridement documents that he or she "performed a debridement of the wound." The patient, like Joe, goes home satisfied and later returns for additional treatments until their wound is fully healed. Medicare is billed for the procedure.

Fast forward a couple of years. The RAC for the hospital's region sends a records request to the hospital, including the aforementioned debridement. Upon

---

[129] An excisional debridement involves the cutting away of devitalized or necrotic tissue. A non-excisional debridement involves the removal of such tissue via irrigation, scrubbing, washing, or other means.

conducting their audit, the RAC staff notices that the word "excisional" is missing from the patient's record. They inform the hospital that the lack of this word means the debridement should have been billed with the code for a non-excisional debridement, which pays much less. In other words, the auditor is saying that too much was paid for the procedure and, given what was documented, a different procedure was performed altogether. Of course, the auditor could have examined the rest of the medical record and easily determined that the debridement was excisional, but that would mean not being able to earn their commission on this recoupment of Medicare funds.

This opens the provider up to what is known as extrapolation. If the RAC in this scenario had audited 100 of the debridement charts and found 25 that were billed as excisional without containing the specific word, then they are permitted to simply assume that the provider made the same "mistake" in ¼ of all of the billings for that service over the entire period under review. Therefore, if the provider had performed 1,000 such debridements, then they would have to give back the difference between the excisional/non-excisional payments for 250 of the procedures instead of just 25. Obviously, this adds up very quickly.[130]

Keep in mind that the audited chart in question could be questioned on an even more subjective level. The auditor might be reviewing, say, pneumonia admissions to a particular facility. In doing so, the RAC may issue a finding that a certain percentage of those patients did not warrant admission to the hospital because they weren't sick enough. While it's clear that a physician at the hospital who has seen the patient, who has become familiar with their history, who has assumed responsibility for that patient's well-being, and who is actively treating them thinks that they need to be admitted, a RAC auditor doesn't need to be worried by such things. If the auditor, who is almost certainly not a physician, deems that the admission wasn't medically necessary, then there's nothing left for the hospital to do other than (a) write the RAC a check for the admission or (b) engage in the appeals process to win back the recouped money from this chart and all the extrapolated charts that followed.

Perhaps this seems strange that a non-physician can overturn the medical judgment of a physician. Sadly,

---

[130] Recent changes to the extrapolation rules have lowered the risk associated with them somewhat. https://www.racmonitor.com/cms-revises-and-details-extrapolation-rules
In reality, these changes have just made the RACs much cleverer in how they attack providers.

this is how payers and their agents work. Naturally, they will claim that they aren't overriding the physician's judgment. It's the physician's fault for not documenting more or the hospital's fault for not properly reviewing the physician's charting.

We hear about defensive medicine in terms of health care providers going to extremes in order to protect themselves from litigation all the time. It's very seldom that anyone publishes a story about defensive medicine to protect against auditors, but this is exactly what happens. Hospitals especially are forced to hire armies of coders, reviewers, case managers, and so forth to guard against recoupment attempts on claims from years past. There is an entire burgeoning field related to Clinical Documentation Improvement (CDI) with seminars, conferences, and certifications all directed to maximizing the amount of information in a chart in the hopes of not just getting payment, but in keeping that payment.

We previously discussed the pressures on a provider to offer patients the correct treatment. Now factor in the possibilities of catastrophic financial failure years down the road for no other reason than an auditing company wants to get paid.

If a recoupment is demanded, there is a legal process to challenge RAC audits. Unfortunately, it features several disadvantages to the provider. First, the money in question could be immediately recouped. Oftentimes, the provider can't just hold on to their funds until the final decision is rendered. Payment is due on the spot. Any time CMS wants money from a provider, the provider really has no choice. If the doctor, hospital, or whoever doesn't have the money available to write a check, CMS simply withholds those payments from all future billings the provider submits. In other words, the provider is seeing Medicare patients for free until CMS is satisfied. Once CMS has recovered all of the due monies, the provider can go back to being paid again. This, of course, can destroy that provider, so occasionally CMS may allow for some leniency, but it suffices to say that the provider is placed in a position of begging for mercy.

Second, when the appeals process is engaged, CMS is in no hurry to allow it to accomplish anything.[131]

---

[131] The process itself involves five different progressive steps following a rebuttal and "discussion period." Essentially nothing happens in the first two steps of Redetermination and Reconsideration. Once these are exhausted, the matter can be taken before an administrative law judge (ALJ), which is where many of the reversals that occur take place. The final level of appeal is taking the case to a United States District Court and having a federal judge rule on the issue.

In fact, the standard appeal takes years to resolve. In 2014, the backlog of appeals was so horrendous that CMS offered hospitals a settlement of 68% of all of their inpatient claims if they would simply agree not to appeal them further. Naturally, hospitals jumped at the chance to recover any of their monies without having to go through the expensive costs of hiring attorneys, consultants, etc. just to gamble on the possibility of seeing their money again. CMS was happy to pocket the remainder of the recoupment with no more questions being asked.

Even after discharging hundreds of thousands of claims with the 2014 settlement, the backlog in 2016 still stood at over 800,000 appeals.[132] Finally, a federal court order in December of that year ordered HHS to reduce the backlog by "30-percent reduction in pending ALJ cases by Dec. 31, 2017; a 60-percent reduction by Dec. 31, 2018; a 90-percent reduction by Dec. 31, 2019; and a 100-percent reduction by Dec. 31, 2020."[133] To HHS's credit, they have been somewhat successful in doing so, with the backlog having been cut down to 444,894 in July of 2018.

---

[132] This includes not only RAC appeals but also appeals on other recoupments from CMS against providers.
https://www.modernhealthcare.com/article/20160209/NEWS/1602 09844/ruling-gives-hospitals-hope-on-rac-appeals-backlog

[133] https://www.racmonitor.com/news-alert-court-orders-hhs-to-resolve-medicare-appeals-backlog-by-2021

That said, HHS has also admitted that it won't be able to eliminate the backlog by 2020, instead claiming that it needed another two years to do so.[134] As part of the same legal proceeding, HHS made a couple of other interesting claims.

When pressed by the American Hospital Association (the plaintiff in the case) to force RACs who exhibited a high reversal rate on their findings to give back their commissions, HHS refused to consider such a measure. Again, we see the government protecting its pets from accountability for poor performance. Recall that RACs are paid on a contingency basis. They have an incentive to issue as many findings as possible. If the provider doesn't have the resources to appeal, the RAC is richly rewarded. If a significant number of their findings are overturned, they simply continue to shoot as many arrows at their targets until something hits. When a proposal was made to hold RACs accountable for shoddy work and a scattershot approach to recouping claims, HHS declined, permitting them to continue with the business model of "throw claims at the wall until they stick."

134

https://www.modernhealthcare.com/article/20180806/NEWS/1808 09936/medicare-appeals-backlog-plummets-more-than-30-since- 2017

The AHA also requested that Quality Improvement Organizations (QIOs) review claims rather than RACs. QIOs are Medicare contractors largely tasked with educating providers and patients on quality of care improvement. The AHA preferred that QIOs review claims instead of RACs because QIOs tend to have actual clinicians on their staff and therefore be more likely to understand why a particular patient was treated in a particular way. HHS, of course, opposed this. Why? Because:

> RACs focus on program integrity and protecting the Medicare trust fund. Taking away more claim reviews from RACs will undermine those efforts, according to HHS. RACs recovered $6.2 billion for the Medicare Trust Funds between fiscal 2011 and 2013. QIOs have recouped $32 million since 2016. In addition, shifting all hospital claim reviews to the QIOs would not be feasible because they don't have the capacity to review as many claims as RACs, HHS said.[135]

Notice exactly what the reasoning is there. RACs are there to "focus on program integrity." Given that there is no "integrity" in anything a RAC does, I must emphasize the second part. "Protecting the Medicare trust fund." Notice then the elaboration. RACs have recovered <u>B</u>illions; QIOs have recovered <u>M</u>illions. QIOs also can't process as many reviews as RACs. In other words, HHS didn't want QIOs conducting the reviews because they don't bring in as much money.

What is lacking from HHS's analysis of the problem?

The simple matter of whether or not the RACs are doing their job correctly. Bringing in clinicians to conduct provider audits would certainly reduce the amount of recoveries. This would hurt the true purpose of the program, which is not to detect fraud or wrongdoing by providers. The purpose of the RAC program is, quite simply, to get CMS as much money as possible by whatever means are necessary. If that means having non-physicians question the medical judgment of physicians, then so be it, as long as the dollars come back into the CMS budget.

---

[135] *Id.*

While the Trump administration has far from a golden record on health care matters, it is to their credit that it engaged in several measures in 2019 designed to roll back the utter impunity and recklessness that has marked the RAC program.[136] Simple, common sense reforms such as holding the RACs to a 95% accuracy rate and a less than 10% overturn rate have proven to be extremely valuable in protecting the interests of providers who want nothing more than to take care of patients, rather than struggling under an avalanche of paperwork just to keep their doors open.

Furthermore, take into account that RACs are just one auditing entity used by CMS to take back payments. Without going into lengthy detail, as that would take an entire book by itself, just know that providers must also be wary of Zone Program Integrity Contractors (ZPICs),[137] MAC audits,[138] cost report audits, the above-mentioned QIOs, and a host of other federal reviews, all designed to strip money away from providers.

---

[136] https://www.cms.gov/blog/recovery-audits-improvements-protect-taxpayer-dollars-and-put-patients-over-paperwork

[137] Normally, ZPICs are claimed to focus on fraud, waste, and abuse. Then again, the "improper" payments sought by RACs are generally classified as waste or abuse as well, so it can be difficult to differentiate their missions sometimes.

[138] Audits directly ordered by the provider's Medicare Administrative Contractor (discussed in Chapter 1).

This, of course, is just at the federal level. There is a whole other layer of regulatory madness deployed at the state level, usually in the name of "safeguarding" the Medicaid program. Since every state has options on how it wishes to implement and control its Medicaid plan, the auditing units vary across jurisdictions. However, as we shall see in the next chapter, the growth of managed care in the Medicaid space has shown that there can be plenty of fraud and abuse that isn't even connected to what physicians, hospitals, and other health care organizations are doing.

For the time being, however, we will examine the activities of some Medicaid auditors to see if they are any less insane than what we have described thus far.

While they have a lot of illegitimate behaviors in common,[139] Medicaid auditors can be even more slippery than those from Medicare. Remember that states have considerable authority over their Medicaid plans without needing federal permission to make changes. This means that states can tweak the rules on an almost arbitrary basis. Provider advocacy groups must remain vigilant in order to stay abreast of these modifications and challenge

---

[139] https://www.racmonitor.com/medicare-and-medicaid-rac-audits-how-auditors-get-it-wrong-2

them as best they can. Still, even when an auditor is demonstrated to be wholly incorrect, the lack of oversight and accountability from state officials leaves them a broad range of latitude in which to wreak havoc.

In one such case, documented by Edward Roche, PhD, JD,[140] the harassment by auditors resulted in tragedy. The provider in question offered durable medical equipment (DME) and counseling services to patients. The provider, acting responsibly, had discharged some bad employees who were engaged in criminal activity. Being criminals, they saw no problem with filing whistle-blower complaints to the state's Medicaid program.

At first, the allegation was that the provider company had no license for conducting its business. After pouring out a considerable amount of money, time, and resources, the provider was finally able to convince the auditor to honor their existing license. As Dr. Roche points out, this should have been resolved with a phone call.

The auditors then proceeded to deny all the claims submitted for payment, escalating its repayment demand to $800,000, plus interest. This was done under the pretense of there being nothing documented regarding the

---

[140] https://www.racmonitor.com/medicaid-auditors-gone-rogue

location of the services provided. Of course, each claim was reviewed and found to have the address for the services appropriately recorded.

The matter continued, with the cost of attorneys, examinations, etc., mounting higher and higher. Each time the auditor was shown to be wrong, they moved the goal posts and declared a new basis for their denials. This health care provider is a family-owned business now driven to the brink of bankruptcy. Two of those family members have committed suicide, and a third has fallen into a deep depression. All of this because of an auditor who (a) must prove that they are justified in having a job, (b) must take a pound of flesh after being humiliated in being shown how wrong they are, and (c) has nigh unlimited power to destroy a provider. This matter, by the way, is still ongoing.[141]

I want to point out something here that I hinted at in the introductory passages of this book. If you are reading this and thinking that these individuals can be challenged because the oppressed provider can contact their representative or senator, you are dangerously mistaken. Understand this: even if the legislator or other official intervenes and corrects the immediate problem,

---

[141] *Id.*

the provider who had the audacity to make such a complaint is now marked for retribution by the auditor, surveyor, or whatever the offending agent's title happens to be. Any provider doing so should be prepared for an endless stream of audits, queries, and manufactured deficiencies for the foreseeable future. Sure, they can continue to make their case to their legislator (or whoever) but the law tends to allow for those sorts of examinations. Even if nothing is ever found, the level of harassment and the constant requests for information can ruin the provider. Eventually, the provider can either file a lawsuit, exposing them to greater expense and future retaliation, or grovel and apologize to the auditor in the hopes that the dogs are called off.

Let us now speak to the commercial insurance carriers and their private war on payment. Surely a private corporation would respect its members enough to streamline their care and deliver on its promises, yes? No. Not even remotely. In actuality, once denials and other administrative delays are factored in, commercial payers take a month longer to pay claims than Medicare does.[142] An Office of Inspector General report in 2016 cited an

---

[142] https://www.beckershospitalreview.com/finance/commercial-payers-take-nearly-30-days-longer-to-pay-hospitals-than-medicare.html

Employee Benefits Security Administration (EBSA) study that found "1.4 billion health benefit claims are filed each year, of which approximately 200 million are denied by plans or insurers."[143] Like Medicare and Medicaid, commercial payers have a crew of auditors always looking for ways to take back monies already paid. However, it would do well to examine some of the mechanisms they use on the front end to make sure the money never gets paid in the first place.

In some cases, commercial insurance companies are very flagrant in denying patients access to care. Anthem, for example, has made national headlines by refusing to pay for CT and MRI scans done at a hospital.[144] This is because hospitals generally have contracts with insurers that provide for more payment for these sorts of tests than the contracts held by free-standing imaging centers. The immediate effect of this policy will be to save Anthem huge amounts of money and to hurt the financial performance of hospitals. Left out of many headlines is the fact that hospital imaging departments are

---

[143] https://www.oig.dol.gov/public/reports/oa/2017/05-17-001-12-121.pdf

[144] https://www.modernhealthcare.com/article/20170826/NEWS/170829906/anthem-s-new-outpatient-imaging-policy-likely-to-hit-hospitals-bottom-line

often the most convenient for patients, with some having very few, if any, alternatives. The ultimate outcome is that access is degraded so that Anthem can make money.

This isn't a new tactic for Anthem. Previously, it had taken the position of refusing to pay for emergency room visits if Anthem determined that the visit didn't meet its definition of emergency.[145] Essentially, Anthem has asked that patients be doctors and diagnose their conditions as emergencies or not. I'm quite certain that most people would admit that there are patients who go to a hospital's emergency department without a real need. I'm equally certain that there are a vast number of people who went to the emergency department in genuine fear of loss of life/limb only to discover that their condition would resolve without serious injury.[146] After a massive outcry and threat of legal action, Anthem amended its ER policy to include certain "always pay" conditions.[147] This is cold comfort to the patients who, while in need of diagnosis and treatment, still can't be sure if their ailment fits in the "always pay" category until they have been

---

[145] https://www.cbsnews.com/news/anthem-among-health-insurers-refusing-to-pay-er-bills-doctors-say/
[146] Id. The article mentions a specific case of a ruptured ovarian cyst and is illustrative of this sort of problem.
[147] https://www.fiercehealthcare.com/payer/anthem-er-coverage-policy-changes

seen by a clinician. Still, just the threat of not paying for the ER bills will assuredly deter patients from seeking care. Even with its softened stance, Anthem gets what it wants, which is cutting patients off from emergency care.

Really, though, imagine just how zealous a payer must be to deny care when it refuses to pay for a gunshot wound in an emergency room. That's how zealous Anthem is.[148]

United has taken a similar approach to surgeries, attempting to block patients from having surgery in hospitals. Instead, United would rather see those patients have their procedures done in ambulatory surgical centers (ASCs) because its contracts allow it to pay less for those facilities.[149] While United claims to be doing this because hospitals are "sub-optimal" and ASCs are "higher quality, consumer responsive and more cost-effective sites,"[150] other evidence paints a different picture.

An investigation by USA Today and Kaiser Health News in 2018 revealed that the push to promote ASCs has come at the cost of patient lives.[151] In addition

---

[148] https://www.ajc.com/news/state--regional-govt--politics/anthem-emergency-room-coverage-denials-draw-scrutiny/sWT8ts3TYv6vNjrEN99kdO/#

[149] https://www.modernhealthcare.com/payment/unitedhealthcare-outpatient-surgery-policy-threatens-hospital-revenue

[150] *Id.*

to finding that ASCs are taking on riskier surgeries and more complicated patients, they found that:

> Some surgery centers risk patient lives by skimping on training or lifesaving equipment. Others have sent patients home before they were fully recovered. On their drives home, shocked family members in Arkansas, Oklahoma and Georgia discovered their loved ones were not asleep but on the verge of death. Surgery centers have been criticized in cases where staff didn't have the tools to open a difficult airway or skills to save a patient from bleeding to death.[152]

None of this is news. Medicare warned about potential deficiencies in ASCs back in 2007, saying that they "have neither patient safety standards consistent with those in place for hospitals, nor are they required to have the trained staff and equipment needed to provide the breadth of intensity of care."[153] Near the close of the USA

---

[151] https://www.usatoday.com/story/news/2018/03/02/medicare-certified-surgery-centers-safety-deaths/363172002/
[152] *Id.*

Today/Kaiser report, Dr. Nancy Epstein, chief of neurosurgical and spine care at New York University Winthrop Hospital, comments that surgery centers doing outpatient procedures on the spinal cord, windpipe, and esophagus is "pretty revolting" and that "Medically, it should not be tolerated, but it is."[154]

Why is it being tolerated? Because payers like United are demanding it, and the patient can either choose to go where their insurance will cover their surgery or go to a hospital that could save their life if something goes wrong and pay for it out-of-pocket.

Now, one might ask how United and its ilk are able to divert patients from one facility to another for a particular test or treatment. This is most often accomplished through the prior authorization process.

If you happen to have a commercial policy, you may have encountered the term **"prior authorization"** **(PA)** at some point. A prior authorization typically takes place when a patient is requiring some sort of test or treatment beyond a basic primary care visit or the lowest level of diagnostics possible (say, an x-ray). It consists of a member of the provider's staff, perhaps a nurse, MA, or

---

153 *Id.*
154 *Id.*

therapist, calling the insurance company and asking permission to perform the test or treatment. This may sound simple, but it is one of the most exasperating experiences a staff member can undergo. A single PA can absorb hours of time just waiting on the phone or waiting for a call back. The call back almost inevitably is accompanied by a demand for more records or more data that the provider simply does not have. Sometimes, it requires another encounter with the patient, forcing them to pay another copay. Sometimes, the process takes weeks. Of course, the patient seldom sees this particular activity as it plays out and perhaps will even think that the provider is the cause of the delay.

On the insurance company's end, the prior authorization is often being reviewed by someone who is not a physician, nurse practitioner, or physician assistant. In other words, as was the case with the Medicare auditors, the kind of people deciding whether or not the treatment or test is needed are not the kinds of people who even have the authority to order the treatment or test in the first place. At best, the reviewer is a registered nurse. This nurse takes the time to review the request from the physician or mid-level provider and will then decide whether or not the more highly trained professional who saw the patient in real life has any business wanting to treat the patient for what is ailing them and whether their prescribed treatment is appropriate.

Once an avenue for denial is found, the provider staff finally gets their call back and starts all the way back at the beginning of the process trying to make sure that the patient's treatment will be paid by their insurer.

There is, of course, an appeals process. This varies with the number of tiers and hoops that the provider staff must jump through, but it almost always ends with a "peer-to-peer review." This is when the doctor or other provider who wrote the order for the patient's treatment finally gets to plead their case to a physician who is employed by the insurance company for the purpose of hearing these sorts of situations. As an employee of the insurance company, the reviewing physician naturally has a vested interest in making sure that his employer is profitable, whereas the ordering physician frequently has none. He/she doesn't own the lab or the CT scanner that will be servicing the patient; they simply need the information from the test to better understand the patient's condition.

While some might scoff at the idea of the insurer physician rubber stamping denials, that is precisely what has been found to happen. In one of the most egregious examples, a medical director for Aetna in California admitted in a deposition that he "never looked at patients' records when deciding whether to approve or deny care."[155] Not only that, but the same medical director said he was just following Aetna's "training" on how to conduct reviews and that, in the particular case being litigated, he didn't even know how to treat the patient's disease. In Delaware, a state Senate investigation found that a contractor for Blue Cross was offering financial incentives to physicians for denying care to patients.[156] In some states, insurers are requiring peer-to-peer conferences to take place within a specific 24 to 48 hour timeframe, even when the initial request is days old, or else they will automatically deny the claim.[157] From my own experience, I can recall numerous cases of our own physicians arguing with insurer doctors over trying to admit or keep a patient in the hospital. The insurer doctor kept stating that the patient simply wasn't sick enough to warrant an admission, several times referring to "criteria"

---

[155] https://www.forbes.com/sites/robertglatter/2018/02/11/former-aetna-medical-director-admits-to-never-reviewing-medical-records-before-denying-care/

[156] http://www.nbcnews.com/id/42613298/ns/nbc_nightly_news_with_brian_williams/t/insurer-denied-needed-medical-tests-senate-finds/

[157] https://www.reliasmedia.com/articles/141921-make-peer-to-peer-happen-within-24-hours-or-face-denied-claim

as the deciding factor, rather than the judgment of the long-time physician with a 10-year relationship to the patient in question and personal familiarity with their problems.[158] Predictably, many of these patients wound up getting sicker, and yes, some of them even died.

I encourage you to ask your own physicians and health care providers about this process. It is present everywhere in the commercial healthcare sector and has been for a long time.[159] There are even YouTube videos showing the entire agonizing prior authorization process.[160]

A study by the AMA shows the depth and breadth of this problem:

> A survey of 1,000 practicing physicians by the American Medical Association, or AMA, found that doctors believe these prior authorizations affect clinical outcomes for 9 of 10 patients. In

---

[158] Several physicians mentioned occasions when they had asked for the "criteria" in question, only to be told by the reviewer that the "criteria" were proprietary to the insurer and so not open for any discussion or transparency.

[159] https://www.cnn.com/2018/02/15/opinions/doctors-take-on-aetna-ford-vox-opinion/index.html; https://www.washingtonexaminer.com/denied-insurers-at-aetna-admit-to-bad-behavior-while-patients-suffer

[160] https://youtu.be/z20wfv4A604

addition, 92 percent of doctors said prior authorizations have led to delays in patient care… The survey found that nearly two-thirds of patients experienced a delay of at least one business day, while almost one-third had to wait at least three business days. The delay can sometimes prompt almost 8 in 10 patients to abandon their prescribed course of treatment, the AMA survey found… On average, doctors are receiving 14 prior authorizations for prescriptions each week, and 15 prior authorization requests for medical services, the survey found. And it takes almost 15 hours -- or two business days -- to process these requests. More than one-third of the physicians surveyed have staff members who work exclusively on prior authorizations.[161]

---

[161] https://www.upi.com/Health_News/2018/03/19/Prior-authorization-insurance-requirements-may-harm-patients-doctors-say/2801521478547/

The comments by a representative of the insurance industry is remarkable in its blatant dishonesty:

> 'Prior authorization is an important and valuable tool to protect patients by ensuring a prescribed therapy is safe and effective for the patient's condition and is a covered benefit,' said Cathryn Donaldson, director of communications for America's Health Insurance Plans.[162]

I am quite sure that there would be very few, if any, arguments about prior authorizations to determine if a requested item is actually covered by an insurance policy. However, by what measure of accuracy can one expect an insurance company's reviewing employee to be able to ascertain if a treatment is "safe and effective" for a patient? As stated earlier, these employees may simply be lay people. They might be nurses, true, but how does a nurse with no connection to a patient (other than having a stack of their medical records) have the ability to veto a treatment recommended by that patient's physician, many of whom have been treating that very patient for years? It is the height of arrogance and presumption for an

---

[162] *Id.*

insurance company to claim it is superior in determining what is safe and effective for patients over the physician immediately dealing with the illness.

Physicians have taken their case to Congress in an effort to pass some sort of reforms to the process. Listening to their comments, you can feel their frustration. Keep in mind, again, that prior authorizations are often directed to tests and treatments that make no money for the referring physician at all:

> "The prior authorization process is out of control. It is increasing and rather than a tool for preventing unnecessary or expensive care, prior authorizations negatively impact my patients' health and is a significant cause for family physician burnout and the closure of small private practices," Dr. John Cullen, a family doctor representing the American Academy of Family Physicians, told the committee.
>
> Dr. Howard Rogers, a dermatologist who owns a small private practice in Connecticut, said his practice spends

70 hours a week on prior authorization. He hired two full-time staff to handle the volume of prior authorizations, costing him $120,000 in salary and benefits that could have been spent on staff education, improved benefit packages for employees and new medical equipment and technology. "One-quarter of all communications in my office, be it phone calls, faxes, emails, EMR notifications, payer portals—they are all associated with prior authorizations, and the kicker is that most of my patients prescriptions and repairs eventually get approved, but only after exhaustive efforts of calling insurers and appealing denials," Rogers said, testifying on behalf of the American Academy for dermatology association.

Dr. Paul Harari, chairman of the department of human oncology at the University of Wisconsin School of Medicine and Public Health and chairman of American Society for Radiation Oncology, explained in his testimony that prior authorization reviewers employed by health insurers are often not in the same specialty are unfamiliar with the condition or prescribed treatment.

Harari pointed out that HHS Office of the Inspector General in 2018 said Medicare Advantage insurers may have incentive to deny prior-authorization requests to increase profits.[163] (emphasis added)

The worst part is that the prior authorization ordeal is just the beginning. Even if the authorization is approved, that just means that the claim is not being denied at this particular moment. There are a host of other reasons for which a denial may be issued later. To list just a few:

1. *A lack of medical necessity*: As was the case with Medicare auditors doing

---

[163] https://wwww.modernhealthcare.com/politics-policy/house-committee-throws-spotlight-prior-authorization-burden

retrospective reviews, commercial payers will often simply claim that a test or treatment simply isn't warranted by the patient's condition, disregarding the medical judgment of the provider who has taken responsibility for helping the patient get better.

2. *The request isn't covered by the insurance policy*: Most people don't read their insurance policies and so have no idea what is covered and what isn't. Many times, insurers will simply claim a procedure isn't covered and hope that the provider and their patient simply go away. Many of them do just that. Sometimes, insurers will misclassify treatments in order to justify the denial. For example, it may say that a weight loss surgery is merely cosmetic and therefore not covered. However, the physician may be making the referral for surgery to correct sleep apnea or

some other disorder. Google will send you to a number of lawsuits based on this sort of argument between patient and payer.

3.   *Coding problems*: We discussed this in an earlier chapter, but coding as a source of denials cannot be overstated. Haggling over what the appropriate code is for a patient's diagnosis or treatment can take months. As the coding system becomes more and more complicated, denials for this reason come more and more easily since there are more areas of potential mistakes on the part of the provider.

The denials can be appealed, with the appeals process regularly culminating in the same peer-to-peer interaction described above. At that point, the patient usually has to become more involved and grapple with the insurance bureaucracy themselves. How difficult is the overall appeals process? Recall the OIG report mentioned earlier with the 200 million claims denied every year. Of that 200 million, less than 1% are appealed.[164]

In considering those levels of review, understand that each one carries a cost associated with it. Any physician or hospital or home health agency or therapist acknowledges the perpetual risk of adverse payer action. To combat this, they hire more staff members, engage consultants, attend educational seminars, etc. all to obtain compensation for the services that have already been rendered or that they seek to render. Every denial means additional staff hours and resources that must be devoted to overturning it. Remember, the provider has already incurred the cost of seeing and treating the patient at some level. The payment they are due will many times not even cover the cost of what has been done. If payments don't come in consistently, cash flow can become an enormous problem very, very quickly.

As we discussed in Chapter 5, administrative costs in the United States far exceed those of any other country in the world. Much of this hinges on the wars that various health care providers must fight in order to get paid and be as secure as possible in keeping their money once they get it.

Let us be clear. Everyone knows that there are fraudulent actors in the healthcare system, just as there are

---

[164] See n. 143, *supra*

in any other industry. That said, there is no other industry with so many levels of review and so much scrutiny from so many different actors as to its performance, nor is there an industry with such a grave significance to the lives of average citizens. I suggest that very little in this system speaks to any sort of true commitment to "accurate information" or "weeding out fraud and abuse" or any of the other payer buzzwords meant to vindicate such a system.

The words of Dr. Rick Boulay, a gynecologist-oncologist, say it best:

> At least weekly, and occasionally daily, insurance companies deny payment for some cancer treatment that I prescribe. In my career, I cannot think of a single aspect of the cancer care continuum that hasn't been denied: surgery, chemotherapy (I once had to cancel a patient's scheduled chemotherapy which was both effective and well tolerated, three months into treatment due to an insurance company refusing to pay for more treatment. They also wanted

their money back for the three previous treatments. In the end, they covered the service), consultations to other medical professionals such as genetics and physical therapy, medications to cover chemo induced nausea, imaging such as CT scans and PET scans. Oh and this is a good one — back billing of a patient's estate for the three grand after she died, for a test to see if the chemo would be effective. It was not.[165]

Ultimately, audits like these, along with the other recoupment mechanisms put into place, are really just ways in which provider compensation can be cut without the political backlash of their being labeled as such. If, say, CMS, knows that it will pay out $1 million of a certain type of claim but that $250,000 will eventually be clawed back for whatever reason it can manufacture, then it has effectively cut the provider compensation by that amount. This is a path of much less resistance than broadcasting a simple, up-front cut in the physician's or hospital's or therapist's pay. The provider might reduce or

---

[165] https://www.kevinmd.com/blog/2017/09/dear-insurance-doctor-not-peer.html

eliminate the service altogether, which means a lot of senior citizens calling their congressmen or senators. Instead, the providers continue to provide the service but just under the threat that, eventually, the dice will come up snake eyes, and they will have to write a check back to Medicare.

It's the same thing with commercial payers. No insurance company wants a story to get out that it is paying less for a particular service. Providers might abandon the carrier's network, or patients might switch to another company. It's much easier to just strip money away from providers on the back end. There are far fewer complaints under such an arrangement, and the provider, with his/her/its pain spread out over the time between audits and reviews, is much more tolerant of the pain inflicted.

A grim assessment of the modern environment was offered by Dr. Roche, in one of his articles for RAC Monitor.[166] The article's main thrust is the new auditor strategy of threatening providers into doing self-audits

---

[166] I cannot overstate the contributions made by Dr. Roche, Dr. Ron Hirsch, and the rest of the staff at RAC Monitor in exposing the corrupt state of affairs in the auditor industry. I encourage everyone to visit their website at https://www.racmonitor.com/. There is a wealth of information there.

and therefore shifting the cost of the work onto the provider rather than doing it themselves. He comments:

> We have lived for years under the Sword of Damocles – the continuing waves of healthcare audits by federal contractors. The names of the Medicare Recovery Audit Contractors (RACs) have changed over time. The program has changed. Some auditors have gone, some have stayed.
>
> But what has not changed is the quality of their work. The coding consultants, attorneys, and statistical experts who help providers through the lengthy, arduous, and very expensive appeal process are familiar with the quality of their work. It can be sloppy, inaccurate, and filled with faults. On average, more than 60 percent of their decisions are overturned on appeal. This means that they are wrong more than half

of the time. But they continue to collect money and even thrive in this protected market.

One might imagine that the auditors' business model is to simply demand repayments from providers, however unreasonable, and then figure that a certain percentage will just pay up without a fight. For the others, there is a carefully managed obstacle course that makes the appeals process difficult and expensive.

This is not to say that there is never some wrongdoing here and there, but it likely is far less prevalent than claimed. And there is no way to fix this chronic problem with healthcare management in the United States. The system is too large and complex to be reformed.

The effects on healthcare providers have been devastating. Year after year, more providers either raise their prices or cut back their services in order to pay for legal and administrative expenses. Some doctors joke that "we spend more time doing paperwork than seeing patients."[167]

These are harsh words describing a harsh reality. They are, however, crucial in understanding the Compromise. None of the people who are making these decisions care about what happens to the patients who are in need of services. Their only concern is in looking good to the Congressional Budget Office (for federal dollars in Medicare), the analogous state body (charged with making the state contributions for Medicaid), or their stockholders (in the case of commercial plans).

As we have hopefully illustrated to this point, it is supremely convenient for the poor, the elderly, and the sicker patients to be allowed to die. Patients are handed over to the Reaper in exchange for cost savings and market share increases. While it can't be done openly, it can be done if the right policy and regulatory levers are

---

[167] https://www.racmonitor.com/medicare-audit-contractors-demand-providers-perform-self-audits

pulled. This is exactly what is happening. In no area is this more obvious than in the case of managed care.

Chapter 8: Why Privatization Never Stays Private (Medicare)

We mentioned managed care briefly in Chapter 1 when discussing Medicare Part C. As a reminder, managed care essentially involved having a private insurance company, known as a managed care organization (MCO), administer the health benefits of Medicare or Medicaid enrollees. The MCO typically works in the same fashion as an HMO. HMOs were extremely popular in the 90s as a way to restrain utilization and keep patient costs minimized. They worked very well at doing so until patients began to notice that they were unable to obtain more expensive treatment or see the physician of their preference. The HMO's control over their access to care led to lawsuits in some states, and a good many HMOs were put out of business as a result. There was even a moderately successful movie, *John Q*, starring Denzel Washington, that was released in 2002 that dealt with a father taking hostages to get a heart transplant for his child because the HMO wouldn't pay for the procedure.

Managed care along the HMO model is rapidly becoming the preferred model for our governmental programs to administer benefits, whether Medicare or

Medicaid. Medicare managed care (also known as Medicare Advantage) enrollment grew 57% between 2012 and 2018, and covers over 20 million seniors.[168] As of now, 38 states use managed care for their Medicaid recipients. This means that over two-thirds of all the Medicaid patients in the country are covered by managed care.[169] Unlike Medicare enrollees, these individuals have no alternative to the managed care system. If they are going to accept Medicaid benefits, managed care is mandatory.

Managed care of government health programs essentially arose out of an admission by federal and state officials that they are not competent to deal with health care matters. As in so many other comparable situations, the decision was made to outsource the management of the health programs to private companies, with the idea that private industry is oftentimes more efficient than the government. Why not let private industry take over Medicare and Medicaid benefits, then?

---

[168] https://www.healthcaredive.com/news/medicare-advantage-is-booming-but-not-producing-savings-report-finds/

[169] https://www.modernhealthcare.com/article/20181027/NEWS/181029950/as-billions-in-tax-dollars-flow-to-private-medicaid-plans-who-s-minding-the-store

On a side note, this isn't to say that Medicare and Medicaid had never used private companies for certain vital functions in the past. We already mentioned the MACs for Medicare in Chapter 1,[170] and states have used private organizations for things like processing payments or accounting measures for their Medicaid programs for many years. Managed care, though, means passing on the entire operations of what had formerly been a government-run enterprise. While the benefits are allegedly required to be equal or better than what is normally provided by traditional Medicare and Medicaid, this supposed equality is a hollow promise.[171]

Recall that managed care typically operates by the MCO agreeing to cover patients for a fixed amount of money paid by the state or federal government per month. For example, an MCO might cover 500 Medicaid patients, with the state agreeing to pay that MCO $100 a month to do so.[172] The MCO will therefore expect to

---

[170] Or "fiscal intermediaries" as they are still sometimes called.

[171] Medicare Advantage plans, for example, offer benefits not covered by traditional Medicare. Most often, these are low-cost items like gym memberships, dental and vision care, meal deliveries, and small discounts on their copays from what regular Medicare would require. Medicaid MCOs have been known to give gift cards to patients for receiving annual wellness exams. While these make for slick marketing, they do the patient in dire straits very little good. For example, see n. 176-177, *infra*.

[172] These values are not meant to reflect real-world rates and are

receive $50,000 a month to pay for these patients' health claims. If the patients only have $40,000 of costs to the plan for a given month, that plan pockets the $10,000 difference as a surplus. If the claims for those patients are $60,000 in a month, though, the MCO has to eat that $10,000 overrun and loses money. It is therefore in the MCO's best interest to keep claims to a minimum. I use Medicaid in the example, but Medicare Advantage operates in essentially the same fashion.

Now, MCOs will claim that they keep claims (and costs) at this minimum because they keep the patients so healthy that the patient doesn't need care. Not needing care means that there are no doctor visits, hospital admissions, and so forth that cost the MCO money. Everybody should be happy with such an arrangement. Unfortunately, managed care typically has a much greater focus on "managing" rather than "caring." Let's consider some general items first and then some specific examples in action.

One of the main differences between MCOs and the standard Medicare/Medicaid program is that MCOs require prior authorization for most treatments and tests. We discussed the horrors of the prior authorization

---

only for the purpose of using round numbers.

process for commercial carriers in the last chapter. It is actually worse in the managed care space. There are a couple of reasons for this.

First, remember that Medicare and Medicaid exist to provide health coverage to older and poorer patients. Statistically speaking, these patients are going to be the sicker individuals in a given population. Since they are the sicker patients, they will have a greater need of services than the population generally covered by commercial carriers. Having a greater need for services means that there will be more requests for different treatments or tests. This means more health care services that the MCO will be asked to pay for. If the MCO is going to keep its costs below its per enrollee payment from the government, it is under much greater pressure to deny as many of these requests as possible, or, at the very least, slow them down to mitigate the damage to its cash flow.

Second, the HMO model itself is more prone to treatment obstacles. Rampant denials were the reason for the collapse of so many HMOs in the 90s. To meet their required budget targets, the organizations were forced to take any authorization for treatment or testing very seriously, with denial as the outcome in mind. MCOs in the Medicare and Medicaid space are no different. Having built managed care on the same foundation as HMOs, it is no surprise that this sort of problem would surface again.

To begin, though, let's just focus on Medicare.

Recently, provider organizations have been begging for some sort of national standards for prior authorization practices.[173] One hospital's director of financial services described the process thusly: "You follow the payer's rules, you think, 'Wow that was an easy process,' you thought you have checked all the boxes to get the procedure paid, only to be denied."[174] She also mentioned the administrative burden inherent in the appeals process, saying that Medicare Advantage plans, on average, required at least three appeals and that successful appeals still took six months to a year to receive actual payment.

Naturally, the insurance representative claimed the clinical high ground for his own as the reason for leaving patients without treatment, with the comment that prior authorizations are "important tools plans use to promote safe, effective and lower-cost treatments."[175] I think

---

[173] https://www.modernhealthcare.com/payment/hospitals-call-overhauling-medicare-advantage-prior-authorization-rules
[174] *Id.*
[175] *Id.*

everyone can agree that the lower cost is a factor. Again, though, there are serious questions about whether or not the typical reviewer of a prior authorization request has the knowledge, skill, or basic concern to decide what is safe and/or effective for a patient.

Granted, speaking specifically of prior authorization denials from such an anecdotal perspective might not be convincing. I concede that I could not find specific data relating to prior authorizations for Medicare Advantage. However, that doesn't mean we can't look at the denial rates in general.

The Office of Inspector General issued a report[176] in 2018 based on concerns that Medicare Advantage plans were doing exactly what any profit-maximizing entity would do in their position, namely, deny claims in order to boost profits. Does any of the following sound familiar?

> Medicare Advantage plans, the popular private-insurance alternative to the traditional Medicare program, have been improperly denying many medical claims to patients and physicians alike, federal investigators

---

[176] https://oig.hhs.gov/oei/reports/oei-09-16-00410.pdf

say in a new report. The private plans, which now cover more than 20 million people — more than one-third of all Medicare beneficiaries — have an incentive to deny claims 'in an attempt to increase their profits,' the report says…

But the inspector general's report underlines potential concerns for consumers. Investigators found 'widespread and persistent problems related to denials of care and payment in Medicare Advantage.' Relatively few people appeal the denial of claims, leaving insurers free to avoid payment. But those who do appeal often succeed. About 75 percent of appeals are successful at the first level of review…

Even as the inspector general's report was issued, on Sept. 27, doctors and patients and members of Congress were expressing concern about some practices of Medicare Advantage plans.

'Patients may be encountering barriers to timely access to care that are caused by onerous and often unnecessary prior authorization requirements,' said a letter sent to the Trump administration this past week by a bipartisan group of more than 100 lawmakers…

When a health plan refuses to authorize a service, the beneficiary may go without it. And when doctors are improperly denied payment for services provided, the report said, they sometimes try to bill patients.

'Some Medicare Advantage beneficiaries and providers were denied services and payments that should have been provided,' the inspector general concluded.

Insurers have for years been accused of similar tactics in other lines of business. 'They save money when they don't provide care,' said David A. Lipschutz, a lawyer at the nonprofit Center for Medicare Advocacy.[177]

When responding to these allegations, the Medicare Advantage plans fell back on the same tired rationale that we heard from their commercial counterparts. "Insurers defend the requirements. They 'protect patients from unnecessary and inappropriate care' and help reduce costs, said Matt Eyles, the president and chief executive of America's Health Insurance Plans."[178] Again, we are faced with the absurdity of remote bureaucrats making determinations about a sick person's health without any real connection to that person's treatment other than what it is going to cost their employer.

In 2017, the National Bureau of Economic Research calculated that Medicare Advantage plans were bringing in around $21 billion in revenue beyond what they were spending on health care claims.[179] This has only increased recently, as the Trump Administration has

---

[177] https://www.nytimes.com/2018/10/13/us/politics/medicare-claims-private-plans.html

[178] *Id.*

[179] https://www.nber.org/papers/w23090.pdf

doubled down on the program with pay increases to the plans in 2019.[180] These numbers make the alleged oversight of the MCOs seem laughable by comparison.

While it's true that CMS has handed out around $10 million in fines to misbehaving plans over the last two years, it is difficult to take those seriously with billions of dollars in excess revenue rolling in and payment increases on the way. Moreover, CMS goes out of its way to hide the fact that a plan has been punished.

Currently, CMS grades Medicare Advantage plans on a star rating that goes from one to five. Highly rated plans are eligible for bonus payments. The star ratings are promoted by the CMS and the MCOs themselves as reliable indicators of how good a plan is. However, according to the inspector general, health plans with serious Medicare violations "can still receive high star ratings" and the bonus payments that go along with high grades. Beginning in 2019, the same report said, "audit violations will no longer be reflected in star ratings."[181]

In other words, a plan might get fined for improperly denying treatment to its members, but that won't stand in the way of that same plan reaping millions

---

[180] See n. 177, *supra.*
[181] *Id.*

of dollars in bonus payments or jeopardize its five-star rating. In effect, CMS is hiding these factors from patients who will then unknowingly hand over their health care to bad actors who have already proven that they cannot be trusted.

Medicare Advantage enrollees eventually catch on, though. A separate report,[182] this one from the Government Accountability Office (GAO), recommended using the number of patients dropping out of Medicare Advantage plans and their corresponding health status as a point of scrutiny. "'People who are sicker are much more likely to leave [Medicare Advantage plans] than people who are healthier,' James Cosgrove, director of the GAO's health care analysis, said in explaining the research."[183] In my own discussions with Medicare patients who decided to switch back to traditional Medicare and away from the tyranny of MCOs, this has always been the major factor. The sicker a patient is, the worse it will be for them trying to obtain health care services.

---

[182] https://www.gao.gov/assets/690/684386.pdf
[183] https://www.npr.org/sections/health-shots/2017/07/05/535381473/as-seniors-get-sicker-theyre-more-likely-to-drop-medicare-advantage-plans

This is well-demonstrated by the attitude taken by MCOs when it comes to patients requiring care in a long-term acute care (LTAC) hospital. LTACs are facilities specifically designed to care for patients who need a very lengthy hospital stay (say, 20-25 days) to recover from a particularly debilitating illness. These are patients who may be on a ventilator for weeks or have significant wounds or infections that are not adequately healing in a standard hospital environment. Of course, this care is very expensive, making LTAC stays almost radioactive to HMO-style payment. Dr. Howard Stein of RACMonitor describes the situation well:

> LTACs have proven themselves to have better patient outcomes then acute-care hospitals in the same areas. However, many MA plans routinely deny authorization for LTAC transfer, saying the same service can be delivered in the acute-care hospital…It is clear to me that some Medicare Advantage plans simply care about the bottom line rather than providing the best care for their members. When patients forego Medicare fee-for-service care for a

Medicare Advantage plan, they are told they will have the same benefits for a lower cost. Is that really true?

Medicare Advantage plans pay for their overhead and generate profit for their shareholders by limiting or denying other services, including acute rehabilitation, subacute rehabilitation, and ambulance transport, just to name a few. Managing cost aims to improve efficiency and quality of care, but payors have crossed the line into withholding care and costs, when possible…

There is little that can be done to solve the problem. I doubt, however, when seniors are recruited by MA plan breakfasts and commercials, they are aware that some benefits just will not be approved. Perhaps they will just be satisfied with the free breakfast and the free pair of eyeglasses these plans pay for.[184]

As one might imagine, there have been lawsuits filed, frequently by whistleblowers. One such case involved a manipulation of patient information that "exaggerated how sick some patients were to boost profits, while getting rid of others who cost a lot to treat."[185] In this instance, the plan kept a list of some "unprofitable" patients that it tried to convince to drop coverage. At the same time "healthier, more profitable" patients were convinced to remain enrolled.[186]

A slew of whistleblower lawsuits hit United on the basis of its Medicare Advantage plan. In one such case, United was accused by members of its own salesforce of deliberately hiding complaints from its members and not properly monitoring employee misconduct, ranging from forging member signatures for enrollment to promising iPads to potential members who stayed enrolled for six months.[187] With all of this flagrant behavior, though, the

---

[184] https://www.racmonitor.com/medicare-advantage-plans-often-decline-authorizations-for-long-term-acute-care-ltac-transfers

[185] See n. 183, *supra*.

[186] This is all against federal law, which prohibits such coverage decisions to be based on a patient's health status.

[187] https://healthjournalism.org/blog/2017/08/lawsuit-claims-unitedhealthcare-concealed-medicare-advantage-enrollment-fraud-complaints/

This article mentions several other lawsuits and references several very good articles illustrating the extensive abuse of the Medicare Advantage program. I highly recommend giving it a full read.

worst part of the story is that "Despite this suit and others…UnitedHealthcare's Medicare Advantage business continues to grow."[188] Whether it's in-your-face marketing, scare tactics threatening a permanent loss of all Medicare benefits for not enrolling in an Advantage plan, or the relentless promotion of MCOs by our political class, there seems to be no slowing the rush to managed care for Medicare patients.

And what is the source of all this non-stop cheerleading by our elected overlords? Why do so many congressmen, senators, and presidents continue to laud Medicare Advantage in light of what we've discussed so far? There are essentially two reasons, both of which are tied to the heart of the Compromise.

One reason is related to the myth that revolves around those talismanic words "quality" and "value." Any applause for Medicare Advantage is almost always immediately preceded by those words, with the usual lack of any definition for what they mean. Without clear meaning, such praise is worthless. This is often coupled with the condemnation of traditional Medicare because it pays on a fee-for-service basis, with the usual lack of any

---

[188] *Id.*

rationale for why FFS is so bad other than "those awful, greedy doctors/hospitals/other providers."

The more relevant reason is that since there are no real objective standards for "quality" or "value" except for arbitrarily defined measures, the praise for Medicare Advantage always shifts over to a discussion of the cost savings that are provided to the Medicare system. Remember the terms of the Compromise. Government officials are happy to turn human lives over to the Reaper if it makes their budget figures look better. The most effective way of doing this is to cut off a patient's access to services. As we have seen, Medicare Advantage plans excel at doing this. The costs that aren't measured in dollars and cents simply aren't important. As long as politicians, policy wonks, and, of course, the plans themselves can claim that there are dollar savings to be had, the applause will continue. If the numbers are shown to be different, then our policy makers will simply find some new way to cut back on access to services and leave patients without care.[189]

---

[189] There is some sign of this perhaps being the case, but the data is far from conclusive.
https://www.healthaffairs.org/do/10.1377/hblog20190813.223707/full/

In light of all of these factors, the federal government continues to double down on Medicare Advantage. President Trump recently signed an executive order[190] on this very point, strengthening the Medicare Advantage program and increasing the plans' chances for profitability. It also forbade HHS from doing anything that would promote traditional Medicare above managed care Medicare. Given the marketing budgets for most MA plans, you would think that they wouldn't need this kind of protection from the executive branch.

There has also been a push to allow Medicare Advantage plans to provide non-health care benefits not covered by traditional Medicare such as supplementary meals or massages. Again, who could argue that these are good things? However, this raises a couple of questions. First, if these benefits are so great, why aren't they covered by traditional Medicare? Probably because the government is trying to make traditional Medicare appear to be an inferior option. Second, what good does it do for the patient to have meals and massage therapy if they can't get diagnostic testing, surgery, or a hospital/nursing home stay when they need it? Of course, it does them no

---

[190] https://www.healthexec.com/topics/policy/trump-signs-executive-order-medicare

good at all, but it does further the goal of restricting access to health care.

Having reviewed the workings of managed care in the Medicare space, let us now turn our attention to Medicaid.

Chapter 9: Why Privatization Never Stays Private (Medicaid)

As mentioned in the previous chapter, CMS has been promoting the shift from traditional Medicare to Medicare Advantage plans, which are structured according to a managed care model. This allows the federal government to hold up its end of the Compromise. Providers attempting to serve patient needs are blocked from doing so by privately-run bureaucracies who are seeking to maximize their profits at the expense of patient care. While ignoring these denials of care, policy-makers get the best of both worlds. On one side, they can wash their hands of the patient and pass off any criticism to the Medicare Advantage plan. On the other side, they can continue to wring their hands and weep crocodile tears over the dilemmas faced by so many citizens that just can't be resolved.

The scenario is no different in the Medicaid environment, except that it is much broader in scope.

Almost 70% of Medicaid beneficiaries are now enrolled in a managed care plan for their benefits.[191] Since

---

[191] You can find a good breakdown of Medicaid enrollment data at https://www.medicaid.gov/medicaid/managed-care/enrollment/index.html

Medicaid is a significant portion (sometimes the most significant portion) of every state's budget, it is natural for lawmakers at that level to want to control costs as well as possible. Since it is so widely believed that private companies handle affairs more efficiently than public officials, managed care seems like a good option. Just from a standpoint of budget simplicity, it is an attractive proposition.

It's also an incredibly effective mechanism for implementing the Compromise.

As was the case with Medicare Advantage companies, the main motivating factor in managed care is money for the plan. Rendering services to patients costs the plans money. Denying access to services makes them money. Medicaid MCOs who claim to save money with lower utilization based on "making their members healthier" are engaged in deception. This promise is usually made to limit their accountability. They can always claim that they just "need more time" to really see the overall health of the population improve. In the meantime, the population starves for care.

Let's consider a few examples.

D'ashon Morris was born premature to a drug-addicted mother in Texas. He had multiple health problems including "bleeding in the brain, internal hemorrhaging, chronic lung disease, developmental delays…a tube to pump nutrients into his stomach, and constant monitoring because his blood pressure or blood sugar would plummet." He also experienced severe breathing difficulties that required a tracheostomy tube to keep him alive. Because of these problems, his foster mother requested the services of a nurse to help provide care. Superior HealthPlan was the MCO charged with paying for these services. Since one-on-one nursing care is expensive, it naturally declined to do so, claiming that there was no "medical necessity" for such a measure.

This decision was made, in large part, based on the determination of Superior's medical director, who had never treated D'ashon and made his determination in contradiction of multiple letters and documentation from the child's actual health care providers. In one instance, during a private phone call, the medical director "'recommended to his other Superior staff that they start communicating with the Dr.'s and try to convince the Dr.'s that the children [with these sorts of problems] do not need the hours that are requested…' Medicaid doesn't allow health care companies to take away nursing hours or therapy without a formal medical assessment and a specific reason, such as marked improvement in health that makes that care no longer necessary."[192]

Once Superior had cut back on D'ashon's care, it then terminated the network contract with the home health agency who had been providing his nursing care, forcing the family to find a new agency for nursing services. This was later alleged to be in retaliation for the nurses' advocacy on D'ashon's behalf. The outcome of all this is predictable.

D'ashon's trach tube eventually came dislodged, and he could not breathe. He coded, and while the hospital that treated him eventually revived him, he was brain damaged. His health problems are now far worse, including seizures multiple times a day. He gets his nursing care one-on-one now.

Some people might say that the financial cost of now having to provide the nursing care is enough of a motivation to keep Superior from doing this to other children. This view is myopic and naïve. First, Superior spared itself the cost of several months of nurse care. The fact that D'ashon is getting the care now is irrelevant. It

---

[192] The bracketed text has been added. The entire story can be found at https://interactives.dallasnews.com/2018/pain-and-profit/part1.html

avoided payments it otherwise would have had to make. Second, D'ashon was probably never going to have a very long life. Now that he is even sicker, he will likely die sooner. This means that Superior will be able to take this large, expensive liability off of its books earlier than expected. Third, it's a fact that many individuals in this position will not make such vigorous appeals or may be lucky enough to have their problems remain stable enough to survive regardless. It is still in Superior's (and other MCOs') best financial interest to deny enhanced levels of care at every turn. The more effectively they can deny, the lower the costs, and the better the cash flow for the company.

You might be expecting this story to end with some sort of punitive measures from the state of Texas. To the contrary, not only were there no penalties imposed, Texas went on to renew Superior's Medicaid contract for $441 million.[193]

D'ashon isn't the only story here. There's also Jose Nunez, the truck driver from Los Angeles. Mr. Nunez was suffering from retinal damage. His MCO delayed treatment for so long that he lost sight in one eye, meaning that he could no longer drive.[194] Ann Carrigan of

---

[193] *Id.*

Iowa requires a special wheelchair to support her head so that she doesn't choke. Her claim for the chair was denied, but the equipment company has provided it to her despite not being paid. The claim for the chair is now in litigation.[195] In Louisiana, managed care organizations' overall denial rates for requests for care were "between 17.0 percent and 18.4 percent," with requests for inpatient care (the sicker patients with a need for more intensive treatment) ranging from "22.7 percent to 23.4 percent."[196]

---

[194] https://www.npr.org/sections/health-shots/2018/10/18/657862337/private-medicaid-plans-receive-billions-in-tax-dollars-with-little-oversight

The article offers several other examples of bad behavior by MCOs: "State lawmakers in Mississippi, both Republicans and Democrats, criticized their Medicaid program last year for ignoring the poor performance of two insurers, UnitedHealthcare and Centene, even as the state awarded the companies new billion-dollar contracts.

In Illinois, auditors said the state didn't properly monitor $7 billion paid to Medicaid plans in 2016, leaving the program unable to determine what percentage of money went to medical care as opposed to administrative costs or profit.

In April, Iowa's state ombudsman said Medicaid insurers there had denied or reduced services to disabled patients in a 'stubborn and absurd' way. In one case, an insurer had cut a quadriplegic's in-home care by 71%. Without the help of an aide to assist him with bathing, dressing and changing out his catheter he had to move to a nursing home, according to the ombudsman, Kristie Hirschman."

[195] http://features.desmoinesregister.com/news/medicaid-denials/

[196] http://ldh.la.gov/assets/docs/LegisReports/2019_04Act710.pdf.

This is a report from Louisiana's own department of health. These findings were apparently not enough to disturb the consciences of the state's lawmakers, as they recently renewed Louisiana's managed care contracts for another term.

The California State Auditor produced an 82-page report reviewing its Medicaid program (Medi-Cal) on the sole subject of "Millions of Children in Medi-Cal Are Not Receiving Preventive Health Services."[197]

California indeed offers perhaps one of the worst accounts of managed care organization conduct and illustrates how the plans are built to restrict access to care.

> Marcela Villa isn't a big name in healthcare — but she played a crucial role in the lives of thousands of Medicaid patients in California. Her official title: denial nurse.
>
> Each week, dozens of requests for treatment landed on her desk after preliminary rejections. Her job, with the assistance of a part-time medical director, was to conclusively determine whether the care — from doctor visits to cancer treatment — should be covered under the nation's health insurance program for low-income Americans.

---

[197] https://www.auditor.ca.gov/pdfs/reports/2018-111.pdf

She was drowning in requests, Villa said, and felt pressed to uphold most of the denials she saw. "If it was a high-dollar case, they tried to deny it," Villa said. "I told them you can't deny it just because it's going to cost $20,000..."

Such concerns are not isolated to one company. Last year, Kaiser Health News reported on similar irregularities at SynerMed, a Medicaid subcontractor that coordinated care for about 650,000 patients in California.

In response to a whistleblower complaint, Medi-Cal said it found 'widespread deficiencies' at SynerMed that put patients "in imminent danger of not receiving medically necessary healthcare services." The company's staffers had falsified documents for years to cover up improper denials of care, according to state officials...[198]

The article goes on to mention other cases of altered records, denied instances of care, and even cases where claims were denied without having been reviewed by the plan's medical director.

These incidents are not a bug in the system. They are a feature.

Similarly to Medicare Advantage, managed care for Medicaid continues to grow. In 2018, states paid more than $300 billion to managed care companies. That was $60 billion more than a decade prior.[199] Much of this increase has been spurred by the Medicaid expansion that was included in the ACA. Even with more and more patients being placed at risk through the denial of access, oversight by state and federal officials remains abysmal. This has led to a lot of calls for investigation, and a lot of public criticisms, but no real action has been taken. Even with the myriad of problems tied to Medicaid managed care, none of the states who have adopted it have seen fit to right their ship and return to administering their own plans.

---

[198] https://www.latimes.com/business/la-fi-medicaid-denial-nurse-20181219-story.html

[199] See n. 194, *supra*.

Why is this? No doubt, the MCOs will tell you that it's because they have done such a great job in taking care of so many patients. However, I submit there is another reason.

When states dismantle their own internal Medicaid system in favor of outsourcing the program to an MCO, employees are discharged,[200] offices are vacated, and entire departments and their budgets are re-organized. It is a structural shift of massive proportions, often done with a sigh of relief, as the state can now rest easy in not having to worry about dealing with a bunch of sick people who don't really pay a ton of taxes and probably don't vote a lot. Once this infrastructure is gone, there is almost no chance of a state having the money, engagement, or willpower to reassemble it. Managed care is therefore a very unsophisticated trap. States walk in with no exit strategy and no real consideration for how this new model will affect patients. Once the reports come rolling in of care denial, lack of access, and refusal to pay, the state officials simply shrug their shoulders and invite the complaining parties to eat cake.

---

[200] Many of whom, by the way, go on to find employment with the MCO.

Many will argue that managed care states always have the option of refusing to renew a plan's contract and replacing any subpar plans with new bidders. This ignores the evidence that the denial of care is standard operating procedure in the managed care world. It simply does not matter which plan it is. Each one, even the "non-profits," are driven by monetary interests alone. States claiming that they can just find another plan that will do a better job are akin to an abused prostitute who thinks that she will find a nicer pimp if she just keeps on looking.

This metaphor holds up on another level. The plans know that the state can't afford to get rid of them. The state has nowhere else to go. Knowing that the state is trapped, the plans can continue to operate with impunity. This entire power dynamic results in a single inevitable conclusion, namely, that the plans no longer work for the state; the state works for the plans. In our experience dealing with these matters, the state will happily concede to its managed care plans as much latitude as they like, with occasional public comments of disapproval that lead to absolutely nowhere.

Recall D'ashon's case in Texas. Not only was the plan not punished, it was awarded with a contract renewal.

States who turn their citizens over to managed care know that they have chosen a one-way door and will expend any and all efforts to squelch opposition or efforts to educate the public on how the privatized system truly works.

And what about those providers who become too much of a thorn in the side of the managed care companies?

They get their contract terminated. We saw this in D'ashon's case when Superior terminated the network contract with the home health agency who went just a little too far in trying to save a patient's life. In more recent news, over one hundred behavioral health providers in Virginia were summarily terminated by the state's managed care networks without cause. Ms. Knicole Emanuel, an experienced health care attorney working on the subsequent lawsuit filed by a group of the providers, has ascribed this purge to the MCOs desire for convenience and a path of least resistance. After all, in her words:

> Since the terminations involved
> multiple MCOs that were not
> ostensibly connected by business
> organization, involving providers

across the state, it became immediately clear that the MCOs may have planned the terminations together. Why are the MCOs doing this, you might ask? If you were charged with managing a firehose of Medicaid dollars, would you rather deal with 100 small providers or two large providers? This appears to be discrimination based on size.[201]

To build on Ms. Emanuel's comments here, it is difficult to conceive of over a hundred providers being eliminated from a network almost simultaneously without there being any sort of coordinated wrongdoing on their part, unless it is a strategic measure by the MCO to save money by destroying access. Think of the consequences of such a move.

First, by curbing the number of providers, the plans automatically lower their internal administrative costs because now they only have to monitor the enrollment and contracts of the handful of those left.

---

[201] https://www.racmonitor.com/exclusive-termination-underway-for-virginia-medicaid-behavioral-healthcare-providers

Second, the providers who are left will be unable to absorb the massive number of patients requiring services. This means that the patients who live in an area with one of the remaining providers will be faced with delays in appointments and treatment. These delays mean that the MCOs will have fewer claims to pay than when the purged providers were still active and submitting their billings.

Third, the claims for behavioral health services will go down further due to many patients simply being unable to find a provider to see them in the first place.

This is the Compromise at work.

I could not get a statement from the Virginia Department of Behavioral Health and Developmental Services as to whether an investigation would be launched into this matter. Even if the providers are victorious in their lawsuit, you can be rest assured that the Virginia government will shrug its shoulders and look the other way.

Finally, we mentioned previously CMS's moves to eradicate the state review of reimbursement rates and their connection to patient access to care.[202] Removing

---

[202] See n. 44, *supra*.

this rule would not be applied to all states equally. It would only be effective in states with over 85% of their Medicaid population having been enrolled in a managed care plan. In other words, states with managed care Medicaid, who are paying billions of dollars to private companies that then withhold care from the poor, would not even be required to report on what sorts of payments these companies make to the doctors, hospitals, etc. who are trying to take care of these patients.

That this is being done for the purpose of relieving administrative burdens is absurd. It is, quite frankly, a sick joke for a state that has abandoned its Medicaid recipients to managed care to then complain about their hardship in having done so. The lack of oversight in the managed care Medicaid space, currently pathetic at best, would be reduced to almost non-existence with this proposal. Meanwhile, the physicians, nurses, hospitals, therapists, etc. who have taken on the burden of actually caring for patients are buried under an ever-expanding mound of paperwork foisted on them by managed care plans who are attempting to avoid responsibility for paying for treatments.

In closing, it is imperative that people understand what is happening to both Medicare and Medicaid.

Commercial insurance carriers are tapping more and more into the administration of public benefits to increase their profits, with the encouragement of our policy-makers:

> The nation's five largest insurers are increasingly dependent on government programs such as Medicare and Medicaid for growth in enrollment, revenue and profits, according to a new Health Affairs study. UnitedHealthcare, Anthem, Aetna, Cigna, and Humana collectively cover 43 percent of the total U.S. insured population, the report said. Due in large part to an aging baby boomer population, Medicare and Medicaid account for nearly 60 percent of the big five's revenues and 20 percent of their plan membership.[203]

As our government pushes more and more citizens into managed care, it pushes more and more money into the pockets of commercial carriers, who then make their

---

[203] https://www.healthcarefinancenews.com/news/big-5-insurers-depend-medicare-medicaid-growth-enrollment-profits

profits based on denying care to the most vulnerable members of our population. When you consider statistics like two-thirds of the growth of insurers like Humana and Anthem since 2010 has been based entirely on taking over previously public insurance programs,[204] this gives you a window into where these companies are investing their resources. As of right now, "Almost 60 percent of the combined revenue of the top five insurers in the United States comes from the government-sponsored health programs Medicare and Medicaid."[205] Revenue from managing Medicare and Medicaid programs went up from $92.5 billion in 2010 to $213.1 billion six years later. Anthem's third quarter profit in 2019 alone increased 23%, almost entirely attributable to its gains in the Medicare and Medicaid space.[206] Any business model that is this lucrative is going to see its masters double down on promoting it.

This is why healthcare payer privatization does not stay private. Privatization is still funded by tax dollars. Even in some of the Medicare/Medicaid-For-All proposals, the entire healthcare system is still being

---

[204] *Id.*

[205] https://www.cnbc.com/2017/12/04/most-of-top-insurers-revenue-comes-from-medicare-medicaid.html

[206] https://wtop.com/business-finance/2019/10/anthem-3q-profit-jumps-23-helped-by-enrollment-gains/

managed by private companies who have nothing more to worry them than their next stockholders' meeting. Privatization is simply an ingenious and insidious way for elected officials to abdicate their responsibility to their constituents. As we have made clear, this gives politicians plausible deniability in the event patients die, providers are punished, or if the overall health of the entire Medicaid population declines.

It's no longer their problem. After all, a deal's a deal.

CHAPTER 10: WHY BIGGER ISN'T BETTER

Thus far, we have mentioned a number of increasing pressures on all the parties who offer health care services in this country. These pressures are there for the benefits of payers and without regard for the patients. Faced with these growing obstacles to both patient care and their own financial livelihoods, providers have reacted in exactly the sort of fashion one would expect when self-preservation is the primary motive. They are combining their forces.[207]

The healthcare industry is going through a historic level of merger and acquisition activity that shows no signs of retreating. The general idea is that creating large blocks of hospitals, physician groups, and other services will consolidate resources (billing, coding, etc.) that will in turn allow for increased protection from payer attacks. Even more so, having more providers under the same umbrella also allows for greater negotiating power against a payer when the time comes for contract renewal. For example, if a hospital can lock down 75% of a given market's patient population as loyal customers, it would

---

[207] https://www.modernhealthcare.com/mergers-acquisitions/hospital-megamergers-continue-drive-near-historic-ma-activity

be extremely difficult for a commercial insurance carrier or managed care plan to try to exclude that hospital from its network.

The rapid push to get bigger and bigger comes at a time when the Government Accountability Office has found that over 80% of the health insurance market in the country is held by three carriers.[208] There is something of a chicken/egg argument as to how this arms race began and who started it. Insurance companies will naturally say that the providers are to blame here and that it was their consolidation that has made such market concentration necessary among payers. While providers certainly aren't blameless, keep in mind what we have talked about to this point. A provider can negotiate as high of a reimbursement as they can, but the decision to pay and the obstacles to get to said payment are largely held in the hands of the insurer alone.

At this point, it doesn't matter who started what or why. There is a race, and it is ongoing. In the course of this chapter, though, we will focus primarily on the providers.

The general logic of economics states that less competition leads to higher price, lower quality of

---

[208] https://www.gao.gov/assets/700/697746.pdf

production delivered, fewer choices for consumers, and higher barriers to entry for newer, more innovative businesses. Highly concentrated markets are known as oligopolies. The end of all competition in a market creates a monopoly for a producer, and the factors mentioned above result in a deadweight loss for the economy.

On the other side of the spectrum, there is the argument that some industries have an organization and scope of goods/services that allow for economies of scale. Economies of scale are the advantages a producer finds that occur when the scale of its production reaches a level when average costs fall as the output of goods and services increase. Perhaps the most famous modern example of economies of scale are the buy-in-bulk strategies employed by places such as Wal-Mart.

There is much debate on where health care services fall between these two concepts. Keep in mind throughout this discussion that not all provider mergers are horizontal, meaning between like providers (as is the case when one hospital system buys out another one). Many take place as vertical integrations, meaning that different levels of services are combined. This was the sort of merger contemplated in 2019 when CVS, a pharmacy chain, completed its purchase of Aetna, an insurance company, for around $69 billion in cash and stock.

Hospitals will argue that mergers act in the fashion of economies of scale and therefore serve to lower costs and produce better care.[209] The greater efficiencies created by the pooling of resources, according to these advocates, allows for costs to be held in check or even decline, while patients are still receiving the services they need. Other parties will take the side of the classical economic argument that competition is preferable to a more centralized marketplace for services.

While the American Hospital Association has released its own report hailing the benefits of hospital and health system mergers,[210] a host of other studies indicate otherwise. These other surveys demonstrate that market concentration of this sort leads to higher prices with little improvement in the quality of care provided. On the other hand, it's also asserted that hospital competition actually increases quality (which is, admittedly, still a difficult term to define).[211] One report from the *New York Times*[212]

---

[209] https://www.healthleadersmedia.com/strategy/hospitals-claim-their-mergers-reduce-costs-disputing-other-studies
[210] *Id.*
[211] https://www.ncbi.nlm.nih.gov/pmc/articles/PMC6170097/
[212] https://www.nytimes.com/2019/02/11/upshot/hospital-mergers-hurt-health-care-quality.html

actually illustrated the same point using physician practices:

> The study found that when cardiology markets are more concentrated, these kinds of patients are more likely to have heart attacks, visit the emergency department, be readmitted to the hospital or die. These effects of market concentration are large.

> To illustrate, consider a cardiology market with five practices in which one becomes more dominant — going from just below a 40 percent market share to a 60 percent market share (with the rest of the market split equally across the other four practices). The study found that the chance of having a heart attack would go up 5 to 7 percent as the largest cardiology practice became more dominant. The chance of visiting the emergency department,

being readmitted to the hospital or dying would go up similarly.

The study also found that greater market concentration led to higher spending. And a different study of family doctors in England found that quality and patient satisfaction increased with competition.

Experts at the Brookings Institute and Carnegie Mellon's Heinz College[213] came to similar conclusions when analyzing industry merger and acquisition activity:

Without effective competition, hospitals can secure higher price concessions in their negotiations with insurers, the Brookings and Carnegie Mellon experts said. Hospitals with fewer than four local competitors are estimated to have prices nearly 16% higher on average—a difference of nearly $2,000 per admission, researchers found.

213

https://www.modernhealthcare.com/article/20170413/NEWS/1704 19935/monopolized-healthcare-market-reduces-quality-increases-costs

As for quality, less competition can lead to worse patient outcomes, especially when prices are set by regulators, as in the Medicare program, according to the paper. Medicare beneficiaries who experienced a heart attack had a 1.46 percentage point higher chance of dying within one year of treatment if they were treated by a hospital that faced few potential competitors, research shows.

When examining the causes of this rapid expansion of health care consolidation, the previously mentioned Brookings Institute report noted that providers are essentially being incentivized or even compelled to make these deals due to the onslaught of regulatory activities imposed upon them:

Providers say they must merge to adapt to changes in federal policy that create a financial incentive for hospitals to control more of the market.

The authors of the recently released paper urge policymakers and enforcement agencies to increase scrutiny of mergers, restrict anticompetitive practices, remove barriers to entering healthcare markets and help independent physicians remain financially viable. Consumers should also be able to access cost and quality data, and providers must accurately identify in-network providers.[214]

Regardless of the cause, the effect is well-known. "Nearly 3 in 4 hospital markets around the U.S. are 'highly concentrated,' according to a new Healthy Marketplace Index report by the Health Care Cost Institute (HCCI)."[215] Whether one thinks this is a good thing is obviously debated by the interested parties, but no one with any honesty can claim that consolidation isn't happening (among both providers and payers) nor is there

---

214 *Id.*

215 https://www.fiercehealthcare.com/hospitals-health-systems/report-three-four-hospital-markets-are-now-highly-concentrated. For whatever it's worth, the same report concluded that "Increasingly concentrated hospital markets have been linked to the rising cost of hospital care by nearly every expert in the field."

any real argument over why it is happening and with such rapidity. Among providers, not only is the pace of merger and acquisition activity continuing with breakneck speed, the participants in those transactions are getting bigger.

> Before 2010, health systems whose revenue was in the ballpark of $750 million to $1 billion were largely satisfied serving one or two cities. Now, those systems are gunning to serve entire counties or even larger regions... Average seller size by revenue grew from $196 million in the first quarter of 2019 to about $597 million in the second quarter of 2019, Kaufman Hall found. That figure reached a record high of $409 million in 2018, according to the report.[216]

This is not limited to mere economic factors associated with lack of competition. Hospitals are also purchasing physician practices and other providers and licensing those entities as outpatient departments of the hospital.[217] This allows for higher billing rates. For

---

[216] See n. 207, *supra.*

example, if a physician's office has an x-ray machine, any x-rays ordered by the physician for a Medicare patient will be compensated by Medicare at a particular rate that is set for physician offices. However, if that same x-ray is performed in a hospital setting, the compensation for the service is higher than the same x-ray from the physician office.[218] To maximize its revenue from a potential physician practice acquisition, a hospital will therefore purchase the practice and then license it as a department of the hospital, even if the physician practice is a long distance away. The hospital will then be able to bill the hospital rate to the payer, and it's compensation for those x-rays will increase above what the physician practice was getting. This, in turn, results in additional direct costs to the patient, as the cost-sharing for the hospital-based tests, etc. will also be more for Medicare patients in the hospital-based setting.

There are currently proposals from CMS to implement "site-neutral" payment rules that will force hospitals to bill for off-site departments as free-standing facilities. Those rules were struck down in federal court

---

217 https://www.modernhealthcare.com/patients/patients-feel-pain-hospital-physician-consolidation
218 This is typically explained by factors such as additional regulatory requirements for licensed hospital space, the presence of potential emergency patients, and other rationales.

and are in legal limbo as of this writing.[219] While it is possible that site-neutral payments will help keep costs down for Medicare and patients, the unanswered question is what this will mean for access to services. The entities being sold are on the market to be bought for a reason. Hospitals and health systems are looking to buy those entities for a reason. "The CMS' payment policies have put the pressure on hospitals to buy physician practices to take advantage of better reimbursement rates for their sites of care, [according to] the Medicare Payment Advisory Commission's staff."[220] In other words, Medicare's own advisory body admits that CMS policies are what drive all this merger and acquisition activity.

If the payment incentives to bill in this manner were removed, would there be enough incentive left for these services to continue to be provided at the physician practice at all? The hospital might simply decide to shutter the x-ray service at our hypothetical clinic altogether, forcing patients to travel to the hospital campus for x-rays. Again, the danger in this sort of direction is that it leads to a lower bill but at the expense of access to patient services.

---

[219] https://www.modernhealthcare.com/payment/judge-tosses-cms-site-neutral-pay-policy
[220] See n. 217, *supra*.

All in all, anyone is perfectly welcome to believe the AHA report and think that the provider consolidation we are currently undergoing is a positive thing. On the other hand, people are also perfectly reasonable in siding with the data that this is a negative trend. I personally find the latter to be more convincing. However, the one thing that is admitted by everyone is that hospitals are seeking additional revenues in order to offset the lower overall margins and compensation that they are currently getting from government payers. Other healthcare organizations are seeking to link up with hospitals in order to find security from regulatory and payment burdens. Nobody appears to have asked what the results would be if these additional revenues are taken away or if the struggling independent group is suddenly blocked off from the safe harbor offered by a larger health system.

As we've illustrated, the problems in healthcare are myriad. Costs are indeed too high, and it's all well and good to seek to lower costs. However, the current proposals seek to solve a problem that has admittedly been created by government healthcare policies driving providers into mass integration strategies. The solutions proposed do not remedy the factors that drove those providers towards such a strategy in the first place. Instead, our overlords wish simply to impose what amounts to a de facto payment cut to provider revenues, likely forcing them to reduce services, and therefore leaving those needing access to services as the odd man out yet again.

Chapter 11: Why Electronic Isn't Efficient

One of modernity's most consistent claims is that, given time, technology will solve all of our problems. This perspective, while sometimes correct, can hardly be regarded as universally true. Anyone looking for evidence of how limited the benefits of technology can be need look no further than the implementation of electronic health records (EHRs) in the United States over the last 15 years or so.

There have been basic computerized systems for medical records going back at least 50 years (depending on how one would define the terms). As electronic methods for charting and patient data evolved, most physician practices and hospitals were slow to adopt such methods for a number of reasons, ranging from a lack of trained staff to the simplicity of paper charting.

This all changed in 2009 with the American Recovery and Reinvestment Act (ARRA). ARRA provided massive monetary incentives for providers who adopted EHRs that met certain standards and allowed for specific sorts of functionality. The official term for these standards was "meaningful use." Providers, naturally, swarmed into the EHR space in order to take advantage of the money being handed out. However, there was also the threat of reimbursement cuts in 2015 (and every year thereafter) for any provider who wasn't using a government-certified EHR in a "meaningful" way. To this day, there are many who have accepted the cut, rather than spend the money necessary to set up a full EHR system. By way of illustration, in 2017, there were still 171,000 eligible providers who were not meeting the meaningful use mandate.[221]

When all of these new computer systems were being marketed and incentive funds were being handed out to those who purchased them, providers of all types were dazzled with stories of how the EHR revolution was going to change medicine forever and for the better. Sales pitches often mentioned how the new system would be more thorough, save time, reduce costs, and increase efficiency. Many were told that the billing changes alone would capture so much missed, unbilled revenue and save so much money that the system would practically pay for itself!

Many providers rejoiced at the brave new world that waited before them. Others cast a more jaundiced eye

---

[221] https://ehrintelligence.com/news/171k-providers-subject-to-meaningful-use-payment-adjustments

at these claims. Regardless, billions of dollars in new EHR contracts were signed, and the hardware and software companies became very, very rich. The initial transition for providers was difficult, but they were assured that with time, training, and habit, the new system would be their best friend. The incentive checks from the government also helped to assuage any hurt feelings or discontent.

Now that reality has set in, let us see how EHR adoption has been going. First, we shall examine the claim that EHRs would reduce costs.

At this point, it would be natural for anyone to claim that providers shouldn't complain too much about the switch to computerized records. After all, didn't the government pay out big incentive checks for anyone who engaged in EHR adoption?

It did, indeed. Billions of dollars in incentives were granted to providers, many of whom used those monies to pay off the outstanding debt of buying an EHR in the first place. Others used it to defray the cost of the lost revenue from the disruption of their practices during the implementation. I'm sure some others used their incentive payments to fund a trip to Hawaii. What all of these different providers have in common is that their incentive money is gone, while the costs of the EHR linger on, and even grow, year after year.

A computer system like an EHR is really no different from any other piece of software. The purchase of the hardware for running it, the training for its use, the integration of operations/accounting/billing, and so forth all require a hefty upfront investment. After that, there is the licensing fee, which recurs for as long as the provider is using the system. This can range from thousands of dollars in a physician practice to millions of dollars for a hospital. Since the incentive payments are gone now, these costs must be directly absorbed by the provider, without any real additional compensation from payers for doing so. Recall our previous discussion of MACRA and similar programs and the physician complaints of having made huge investments in technology in order to meet the reporting mandates. Recall as well how the return on investment for doing so was negligible. At this point, "the cost of software and implementation are inhibiting growth from being more robust."[222]

Moreover, the cost increases don't end there.

---

[222] https://www.healthcarefinancenews.com/news/ehr-investments-slowing-down-hospitals-cite-high-costs-study-finds

A study published in the *Journal of the American Medical Association* indicated that EHR adoption had done nothing to improve administrative costs. The basic conclusion was that, since providers must deal with multiple payers, all of whom have different IT systems themselves, different policies, different standards, and different payment rates, healthcare EHRs simply cannot keep up.

> Costs associated with billing were even higher when researchers took the cost of the EHR software into account, rising to $32.52 for a primary-care visit and $319.80 for an inpatient surgical procedure. Across the types of patient encounters, billing costs made up between 3.1% (inpatient surgery) and 25.2% (emergency department visit) of professional revenue.

> "These findings suggest that significant investments in certified health information technology have not reduced high billing costs in the United States," the researchers wrote.

The researchers could not attribute the high costs to "any significantly wasteful or inefficient efforts" in billing, something they speculate could be due to the fact that the health system uses a single billing organization. Instead, they attribute the costs to differing contracts with payers and price schedules that remain unstandardized.[223]

Not only did the EHR not lower costs, it actually increased the costs in question. In a very sad comment towards the end of the article here, one of the authors expressed their hope that the study results would be a "wake-up call" and that the focus could shift to "administrative simplification." Anyone reading this book up to this point should understand by now that "administrative simplification" is not going to happen in any meaningful way because complexity is how the Compromise thrives. Burying a provider under an endless sea of regulations and back-end costs is effective at killing access and doing so in a way that the average

---

223

https://www.modernhealthcare.com/article/20180220/NEWS/180229998/ehrs-do-not-lower-administrative-billing-costs-study-finds citizen/voter will not notice or understand. Recall Mr. Gruber's comments about the advantages of no transparency. Opacity is the goal.

This is confirmed by a 2016 survey by Deloitte that concluded that:

> The majority of physicians…hold relatively negative perspectives on some aspects of EHRs, and this has not improved since our last survey in 2014. Indeed, three out of four physicians believe that EHRs increase practice costs, outweighing any efficiency savings, and seven out of 10 physicians think that EHRs reduce their productivity. Moreover, physicians are less likely to think that EHR capabilities support clinical outcomes than they did in the 2014 survey.[224]

The survey tries to mitigate this enormous dissatisfaction by claiming victories for the EHR initiative in that three in five physicians wouldn't change their

---

[224] https://www2.deloitte.com/us/en/pages/life-sciences-and-health-care/articles/health-care-current-september27-2016.html

existing EHR and 78% find them valuable for "analytics and reporting." The survey doesn't expound on these points very much, but I'm fairly confident that, if the questions had dug a bit deeper, they would have found that the root cause of these numbers are easily explained.

First, no physician wants to change EHRs because they are basically trapped. They spent a huge amount of money, time, and other resources to engage with the system they have. Spending thousands of dollars more and suffering through the massive disruption in their practice (and cash flow) that a second implementation would bring is a nightmarish scenario. The time to educate themselves and their new employees alone would not be worth the agony of a switch, so the physicians stay shackled to their existing EHR vendor and hope they can make the best of the bad situation.

Second, the physicians who say that EHRs work well in reporting and analytics are absolutely correct. Most EHRs do those things quite well. That's a good thing, too, since, as we've discussed in Chapter 4, the reporting requirements being imposed on health care providers are a vital part of ever-increasing administrative costs rampant in healthcare policy-making. Notice again that the providers are trapped. They have been forced to purchase computer systems so that they can be forced to comply with reporting measures. The only real way to escape the rules is to stop taking patients who have payers that mandate such things. Initially, this means no CMS patients, but it is expanding rapidly into the commercial space.

It's natural then for physicians to want to keep their EHRs. They have no other way of reporting the data that is required from them. Giving up the EHR would mean first taking the cut from CMS for not having one and then taking the second cut for not being able to report all the required measures. It remains astonishing that CMS was able to compel providers to buy tools to do the extra work that CMS forced them to do.

Since we can all agree that EHRs do reporting and analytics well, what about the things that actually matter for patient care? Have EHRs produced better patient outcomes?

For this topic, I direct you to a Kaiser report entitled "Death by a Thousand Clicks."[225] While a significant portion of the article consists of a litany of patient deaths and tragedies, it can be best summarized by these two paragraphs:

---

[225] https://khn.org/news/death-by-a-thousand-clicks/

But 10 years after President Barack Obama signed a law to accelerate the digitization of medical records — with the federal government, so far, sinking $36 billion into the effort — America has little to show for its investment. KHN and Fortune spoke with more than 100 physicians, patients, IT experts and administrators, health policy leaders, attorneys, top government officials and representatives at more than a half-dozen EHR vendors, including the CEOs of two of the companies. The interviews reveal a tragic missed opportunity: Rather than an electronic ecosystem of information, the nation's thousands of EHRs largely remain a sprawling, disconnected patchwork. Moreover, the effort has handcuffed health providers to technology they mostly can't stand and has enriched and empowered the $13-billion-a-year industry that sells it...

Quantros, a private health care analytics firm, said it has logged 18,000 EHR-related safety events from 2007 through 2018, 3 percent of which resulted in patient harm, including seven deaths — a figure that a Quantros director said is "drastically underreported."[226]

The government spent $36 billion and imposed its will upon the health care industry in order to force people with a mission for treating sick people to buy computers that have led to physician burn-out, nurse alert-fatigue, billing abuses, patient harm, and networks of EHRs with no interoperability whatsoever. Let's not forget the higher costs as well. What the government got in return was access to vast amounts of patient and provider information that it previously did not have. There isn't much else positive in the deal to speak of (assuming you can call this much information in the hands of the government a positive thing).

Naturally, the article paints this inventory of blown expectations as just poor execution of a well-intentioned idea. Whether it is or not, it has made for a

---

[226] *Id.*

cataclysmic change in health care from which there is literally no return in the current atmosphere of punishing providers who do not follow the government demands in lock-step.

Dr. John Prunskis, MD, made reference to this in an interview saying, "If this system was so good, then tell me, when was the last time the government paid you to do something? It's impressive, the lobbying efforts of the EMR companies, to ram this flawed system onto the American healthcare community."[227]

While the problem of EHRs might seem to stand alone from the other problems mentioned in this book, they actually interact quite a bit.

> The Centers for Medicare & Medicaid Services' (CMS) 1995 and 1997 updates to documentation guidelines for evaluation and management, which have been widely adopted by third-party payers as the standard for proper patient documentation, play a major role in most physicians' stress from

---

[227] https://www.mdmag.com/medical-news/why-are-emrs-so-terrible

excessive note-taking, [Rep. John] Fleming (R-LA) said. He pointed to other elements of modern documentation standards, such as required preauthorization and precertification via paperwork for supplemental tests and evaluations that only add to that burden.

On top of system difficulties leading to physician stress, patients and consumers may eventually bear the burden of cost from health care facilities' expenses on information technology, Fleming said. "If you assume more than 50% of time is spent on administrative work and doesn't require a license to do it, that accounts for a huge amount of pent-up activity, and that's very inefficient for the system," Fleming said. "It's no wonder the costs for health care have gone up how they have."[228]

It's no wonder at all.

---

[228] *Id.*

It really doesn't matter if the provider is small or large in this case. You might have less than 100 beds like Western Missouri Medical Center[229] or a nationally-renowned cancer center like MD Anderson.[230] You could be the IT director or the Chief Medical Information Officer at Shriners Hospital for Children. You could be one of the 1,250 physicians who participated in a Mayo Clinic study that found that "Electronic health record systems score in the bottom 9th percentile of technologies when evaluated for usability…That's a problem, because physicians who rate their EHR experience poorly are more likely to report symptoms of burnout, study authors wrote."[231]

Whatever your role or position, you know by now that the hallmarks of EHRs are their burden on providers, their ability to cripple any size organization financially, and their "failure to fulfill the promise."[232]

---

[229] https://ehrintelligence.com/news/cerner-implementation-at-mo-hospital-causing-billing-problems

[230] https://www.beckershospitalreview.com/finance/md-anderson-points-to-epic-implementation-for-77-drop-in-adjusted-income.html; https://www.modernhealthcare.com/article/20170106/NEWS/170109948/md-anderson-cancer-center-to-cut-900-jobs-due-to-losses-from-ehr-rollout

[231] https://www.modernhealthcare.com/information-technology/physicians-score-ehrs-f-usability-study-finds

[232] https://www.beckershospitalreview.com/healthcare-information-technology/shriners-hospitals-for-children-cmio-dr-

Regardless of the overwhelming evidence of how the "tech revolution" has failed in medicine to this point, we are still fed a constant diet of propaganda insisting that it has been a resounding success. Naturally, the government wants people to believe that its $36 billion was well-spent. EHR companies want to continue to market their wares. Hospitals and providers want to put on a happy face because nobody wants to admit that they are delivering care with this gigantic anchor weighing down their overall ability to perform at a high level.

The reality is quite different. Every time you hear about new reporting requirements or "quality" measures, what you are actually hearing is the government doubling down on the electronic health record. Every one of these measures is another chain tying health care providers to their EHR because there is no other way for them to pull, process, and transmit all this data to the mandated specifications.

There is one other matter to consider here as well. In the past, if any person wanted to illegally access the medical records of a patient, the prospective snoop would have to break into the physical location housing the records, find the records in question, and then copy them or otherwise make off with whatever it is they were after. With the modern EHR, all you need is a good hacker.

With all of this personal medical and financial information available in one location now, hackers are increasingly focusing on healthcare organizations for cyber-attacks. "Beazley Breach Insights found that healthcare is the industry most targeted by cyber criminals, accounting for 41 percent of all breaches reported to the firm last year."[233] This, of course, places all of this patient data at risk, but there's more to it than that. Like everything else that revolves around EHRs, the risks associated with potential hacks come with a cost. "Health providers will spend an estimated $408 per each lost or stolen patient record--about three times more than other sectors."[234]

In other words, a particular method for record storage (the EHR) was made compulsory. This method is, by definition, more vulnerable to piracy by bad actors. Providers saddled with the compulsory regulations have been left to fend for themselves to protect their patients from these bad actors, without a single cent of additional compensation to help pay for defense. Instead, it's just

---

[233] https://www.healthcarefinancenews.com/news/hospitals-face-rising-risk-sophisticated-cyberattacks
[234] *Id.*

one more cost they have to absorb from an ever shrinking and ever more slippery pool of compensation.

So when you hear about the wonders wrought by electronic health records or hear politicians patting themselves on the back for enabling this fiasco, just remember that they have no interest in telling you the truth. Don't believe the hype.

Chapter 12: Miscellaneous Myths

Any work like this could go on almost forever. There are literally hundreds of thousands of pages of federal regulations. Some affect health care directly, others only indirectly. This doesn't even begin to touch on the variant state regulations and the wildly differing policies and rules among payers. Knowing that we have to close out our work at some point, this chapter will be a synopsis of a few major myths that are still perpetrated throughout American society, usually by promoters of the Compromise, in order to distract the populace from what actually lies at the core of the health care industry's problems. This chapter is essentially to give you enough information to refute this nonsense when you hear it so that you can move on to a hopefully more productive conversation.

1.   **<u>End of Life Care is really what drives the high cost of medical care in the United States.</u>**

This is frequently tossed about as the "real" problem with American healthcare. Typically, you hear this myth as some generalized statement about how old people are the issue, with "the last 6 months of health care services cost more than all the other health care services from the rest of a person's life combined." Sometimes, this will even be floated by proponents of euthanasia in order to sell that as the cure for what ails the system. Almost always, though, this is what is cited as being the true culprit behind health care costs. If only we could curtail the expenses associated with end of life care, so the story goes, health care costs would decrease into "normal" ranges.

Is this borne out by the available data, though?

We first direct your attention to a 2015 study published in the American Journal of Public Health by Drs. Melissa Aldridge and Amy Kelley.[235] They reviewed the total healthcare expenditures for the United States in 2011. This amounted to around $1.7 trillion. They likewise identified the top 18.2 million of individuals whose healthcare costs comprised the top 5% of those expenditures. The study then subdivided the high cost group into three categories:

- individuals who have high healthcare costs because it is their last year of life
- individuals who experience a significant health event during a given year but who return to stable health, and

---

235 https://www.ncbi.nlm.nih.gov/pmc/articles/PMC4638261/

- individuals who persistently generate high annual healthcare costs owing to chronic conditions, functional limitations, or other conditions but who are not in their last year of life and live for several years generating high healthcare expenses.[236]

Their conclusions run quite contrary to the standard narrative of how much of healthcare spending is actually being directed to end of life concerns. Ultimately, they found that end of life care only comprises around 13% of that $1.7 trillion dollar figure above. Of those 18.2 million people in the high cost cohort, a mere 11% were in the last year of their lives.[237]

The largest population in the high cost group were actually those in the second category. These are people who suffered a discrete healthcare event—say, a heart attack—but went on to recovery and stability afterward. This group was 49% of the high cost individuals.

The remaining high cost individuals (40%) were those with persistent high costs, typically due to chronic conditions or other similar factors. According to the study, this is the group most likely to benefit from health

---

[236] *Id.*

[237] Or 80% of the total deaths in 2011.

care interventions and therefore be the greatest area for potentially lowering costs.

With that in mind, why is there so much focus on end of life care? If someone showed you the following diagram (which is part of the Aldridge/Kelley study), would you immediately assume that end of life care is the real problem that warrants such a disproportionate focus?

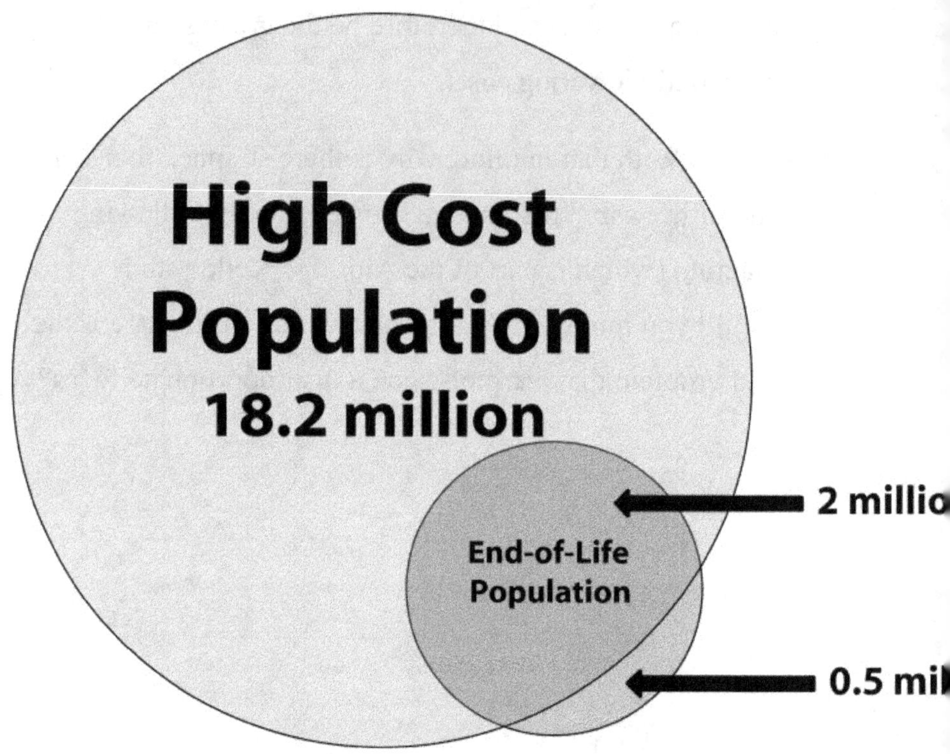

I doubt that you would. Your more likely response would be, "End of life care might be something to look at, but it's obviously not the major issue here."

Further evidence that end of life care is far from the worst of our problems came in a 2018 study[238] that examined just how well the healthcare industry performs in predicting what patients will die and when. After all, for the End of Life Care myth to have any credibility, we must be able to accurately predict what patients will die

---

[238] https://science.sciencemag.org/content/360/6396/1462

so that the "wasteful" healthcare spending engaged in the fruitless efforts to keep them alive can be restrained, cut off, or whatever other strategy proponents of the Myth wish to use.

The study opens with commentary from a couple of myth peddlers:

> For example, an article in the *New Yorker* states that "…for most people, death comes only after long medical struggle with an incurable condition—advanced cancer, progressive organ failure…, or the multiple debilities of very old age. In all such cases, death is certain, but the timing isn't." Likewise, the *New York Times* asks, "Does it make sense that older adults in their last year of life consume more than a quarter of Medicare's expenditures…? Are there limits to what Medicare should spend on a therapy prolonging someone's life by a month or two?"[239]

---

[239] *Id.*

As we discussed above, there are a lot of people who suffer from discrete health events who recover in spite of terminal predictions. There are also people with chronic health conditions who live long lives with high levels of healthcare spending outside of their last year/six months of life. The main issue then is that "Those who end up dying are not the same as those who were sure to die."[240] How is a measure of "wasteful" end of life spending supposed to be measured, then?

The study used machine learning algorithms to plot the mortality of a random sample consisting of 20% of Medicare enrollees. What they found is that less than 5% of the spending involved is accounted for by those with a predicted mortality rate of 50% or more. In other words, if there is a "problem," it isn't with end of life care. It's with the amount of money spent on anyone who happens to be very sick. Some may recover and some may not, but they will all see a high level of healthcare spending due to their condition:

> In sum, although spending on the
> ex post dead is very high, we find
> there are only a few individuals for
> whom, ex ante, death is near

---

[240] *Id.*

certain. Moreover, a substantial component of the concentration of spending at the end of life is mechanically driven by the fact that those who end up dying are sicker, and spending, naturally, is higher for sicker individuals. Of course, we do not—and cannot—rule out individual cases where treatment is performed on an individual for whom death is near certain. But our findings indicate that such individuals are not a meaningful share of decedents.[241]

This takes us back to the Aldridge/Kelley study. The dollars spent on end of life care are not where the significant cost lies. That is instead primarily distributed among the population with specific health events from which they recover and among those with chronic ailments or disabilities. As we learned in Chapter 4, there is only so much influence that a medical care provider can have over these sorts of patients. Health is primarily dictated by individual choices, social factors, and

---

241 *Id.*

genetics. Any conceivable interventions should be directed at those matters and not from trying to target an arbitrary date at which we feel death is imminent so that we begin curbing treatment.

The Compromise, as usual, wants us to focus on access to care and denying treatment to the infirm. It would be much easier for Medicare to not pay for these treatments and keep that money. Likewise, politicians have found an easy scapegoat with a limited constituency. After all, how many dead people will be around to vote against them? Patients are beginning to buy into this lie as well. It is, of course, far, far more convenient for a patient to accept death as an inevitability and to continue to smoke, eat what they want, etc. than it is to consider real changes to their lifestyle in accordance with their physicians' instructions.

In summation, there is a sick person problem rather than a dying person problem. Focusing on the latter is just a clever way of being duped into thinking that access to care and treatment is a burden on the system.

2.   **<u>If the United States spent as much as other countries on other social programs, its healthcare spending wouldn't be so out of control.</u>**

This myth revolves around the idea that the United States doesn't have the same entitlement program infrastructure as other nations, and, if it did, healthcare costs would be effectively checked. Essentially, more money spent in the United States for schools, day cares, and social programs would mean a healthier population, which would then reduce healthcare expenditures. The corollary to this view is that the investment in these other social services to be effective would be less than what is being spent on healthcare. The increased spending would therefore still be a net gain for the country due to the healthcare savings.

As usual, however, this conventional wisdom runs contrary to the evidence we have on-hand.

A study published in 2019 entitled "The Relationship Between Health Spending And Social Spending In High-Income Countries: How Does The US Compare?"[242] examined this precise issue. First, it looked at the social services expenditures across various OECD[243] countries. In defining "social services," the authors stated:

242

https://www.researchgate.net/publication/335183812_The_Relatio nship_Between_Health_Spending_And_Social_Spending_In_High-Income_Countries_How_Does_The_US_Compare

[243] Organization For Economic Cooperation and Development

We defined social spending as countries' expenditures on social programs. As social spending is thought to influence health care spending through its impact on health out-comes, we focused on spending related to social programs that influence the key determinants of health. This led us to focus on spending related to active labor-market programs (such as welfare-to-work programs), incapacity and unemployment benefits, family programs, housing, pensions, and education.[244]

In comparing the US specifically with the rest of the OECD, the study found that the United States actually spent more on social services than the OECD average as a percentage of its GDP. As the diagram below indicates, while not spending as much as Denmark, the US ranks higher in this category than Canada or Israel and is in line with the percentages spent by Japan, Australia, and Iceland.

------

[244] See n. 242, *supra*.

Percent of gross domestic product (GDP) devoted to social spending and health care spending in the US and other Organization for Economic Cooperation and Development (OECD) countries

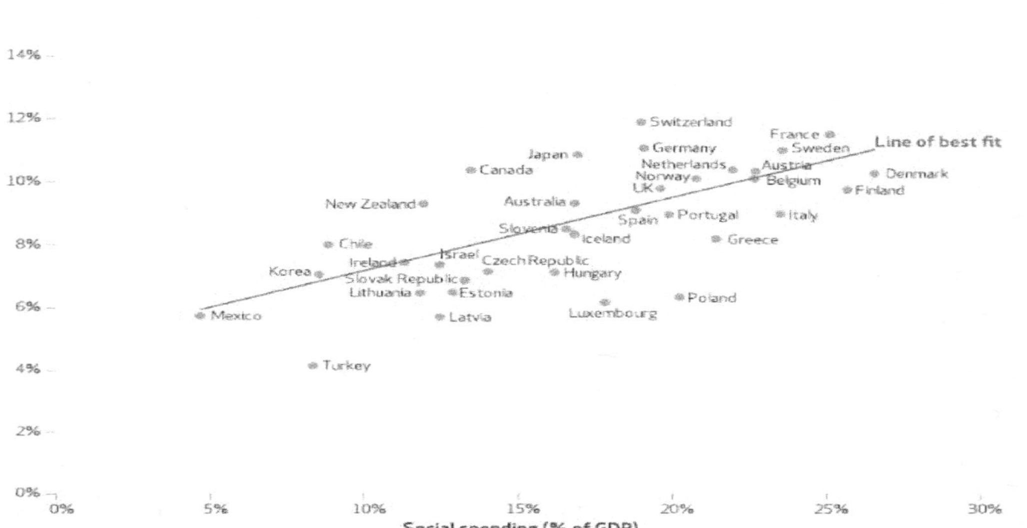

However, even with this level of parity, and even with comparable increases in social spending across the US and other nations from 1980 to 2015, America is still spending far more on healthcare than these other countries. Moreover, across all countries, those that spent more on social services tended to be in the same group who spent more on healthcare. [245]

Nothing in this data should be construed as saying that spending money on social services is bad, that America can't spend its money on social services better, that spending less on social services is somehow desirable, or that spending more on social services would not help. What it does mean is that it is wrongheaded to make blanket statements about how the US should follow the path of other countries who spend more on social services and therefore spend less on healthcare. This is becoming a critical part of the national healthcare conversation, as more and more focus is being placed on the social determinants of health with the expectation that doctors, hospitals, and other providers should intervene in those areas without any compensation for doing so.

---

[245] *Id.*

3. **<u>Medical errors are the third leading cause of death in the United States.</u>**

Most of us are familiar with this myth because it is repeated ad nauseam in movies, television programs, novels, and other works of fiction. I still remember the first time I heard it paraphrased in such a medium. It was Andre Braugher in the pilot commercial for his otherwise quite good (yet short-lived) show, *Gideon's Crossing.*

At the time, I was new to concepts of how healthcare worked. The claim was so outrageous that I figured that it had to be true. Surely, nobody could just fabricate such a statistic.

As I got deeper into healthcare, I found that the claim was essentially a summary of a 1999 report entitled, "To Err Is Human: Building A Safer Health System."[246] The basic point of the report is that, conservatively, 44,000 people die every year due to medical errors in hospitals alone. The more accurate number, according to the authors, may be closer to twice that number.[247] Naturally, the study focuses on the catastrophic human cost of so many untimely deaths. It also, however, discusses how costly these alleged errors are to the healthcare system overall. It estimated that just the cost of

---

[246] https://www.ncbi.nlm.nih.gov/pubmed/25077248
[247] https://www.ncbi.nlm.nih.gov/books/NBK225179/

adverse drug events for inpatients was likely $2 billion a year.

"To Err Is Human" was later followed up by two other papers, one in 2013[248] and the other in 2016,[249] that inflated the mortality numbers even more. The latter of these papers gave rise to the ubiquitous phrasing of medical errors as the "third leading cause of death" in the country. Now, we are led to believe that the number of preventable deaths caused by medical errors--physician and hospital mistakes--are somewhere between 251,000 and 440,000 deaths annually.

If one accepts these figures, it's easy to see why the push for "value" and "quality" has had so much traction. After all, it's obviously hospitals and doctors who are screwing up, killing patients, and making the system cost so much with their recklessness. If only such screw-ups could be eliminated, the reasoning goes, lives would be saved and costs would go down. This then serves as the justification for a multitude of punishments and penalties inflicted on health care providers for supposed mistakes. As we've already covered, though, the "errors" that are targeted by government policy typically

---

248

https://journals.lww.com/journalpatientsafety/Fulltext/2013/09000/A_New,_Evidence_based_Estimate_of_Patient_Harms.2.aspx
249 https://www.bmj.com/content/353/bmj.i2139

(1) are not within the providers' control, (2) are not germane to patient care, (3) are completely absurd in their construction, (4) harm patient outcomes, and most especially (5) make it more difficult for services to be provided, killing access to treatment for current and future patients.

As noted throughout this book, this approach is misguided even if the statistics are true. If the statistics are not true, you have one more piece of evidence that the approach isn't misguided, but rather malevolent.

So what about the "To Err Is Human" report itself?

First, let's consider the estimates of the report itself. If the numbers presented therein are true, then, as one critique points out, more Americans are killed in hospitals every six months than died in the entirety of the Vietnam War.[250] We would think that most people, upon hearing such a comparison, would immediately be suspicious of whomever performed those calculations. Recall that the "To Err Is Human" estimates are on the low end amongst the reports we mention here. If we accept the high end estimates, more people die in hospitals in a single year than died in the whole course of fighting World War II. To put it in even more concrete

---

[250] https://jamanetwork.com/journals/jama/fullarticle/194039

terms, there are around 700,000 deaths of hospital patients per year.[251] These statistics would have you believe that anywhere from *one-third to over one-half* of all of these deaths are due to preventable errors.

Perhaps this seems realistic to you. If so, I direct you to three reports that were released in the aftermath of "To Err Is Human."[252] They all point out various problems with the study as it relates to its statistical modeling. To summarize, there are serious problems with items ranging from how a medical error is defined to how a death is allegedly connected to the alleged error to how one counts those and attempts to extrapolate the number across the entire country. While these ripostes to the enormous mortality numbers presented are worth examining in their own right, let us instead focus on a 2001 New England Journal of Medicine article by Dr. Troyen A. Brennan, M.D., J.D., M.P.H. Dr. Brennan's opinion is significant because he served as an author on both the primary studies that serve as the backbone of the "To Err Is Human" calculations.

---

[251] See n. 258, *infra*.

[252]

http://citeseerx.ist.psu.edu/viewdoc/download?doi=10.1.1.593.586 5&rep=rep1&type=pdf; http://ecp.acponline.org/novdec00/sox.htm; https://jamanetwork.com/journals/jama/fullarticle/194039

In his article, "The Institute of Medicine Report on Medical Errors — Could It Do Harm?",[253] Dr. Brennan takes exception to the idea that hospitals are killing up to 98,000 people a year. He begins by noting the problem with defining what a medical error might be. Recalling his work on the prior studies, he states:

> [W]e agreed among ourselves about whether events should be classified as preventable or not preventable, but these decisions do not necessarily reflect the views of the average physician and certainly do not mean that all preventable adverse events were blunders. For instance, surgeons know that postoperative hemorrhage occurs in a certain number of cases, but with proper surgical technique, the rate decreases. Even with the best surgical technique and proper precautions, however, a hemorrhage can occur. We classified most postoperative hemorrhages resulting in the

---

[253] https://www.nejm.org/doi/full/10.1056/NEJM200004133421510

transfer of patients back to the operating room after simple procedures (such as hysterectomy or appendectomy) as preventable, even though in most cases there was no apparent blunder or slip-up by the surgeon. The IOM report refers to these cases as medical errors, which to some observers may seem inappropriate.[254]

Even after admitting that some may charge this sort of criticism as "hairsplitting," Dr. Brennan goes on to mention four other aspects of the report that should give anyone pause in accepting its findings as dogmatic.

A. "First, the report and the accounts of it in the media give the impression that doctors and hospitals are doing very little about the problem of injuries caused by medical care…[I]f one extrapolates from our studies in New York and in Colorado and Utah in order to

____

[254] *Id.*

calculate the number of deaths nationwide due to substandard care, the total decreases from 92,000 deaths in 1984 (on the basis of the data in New York) to 25,000 in 1992 (on the basis of the data in Colorado and Utah). Although no statistician would be convinced by data extrapolated from three different settings, and although my colleagues and I have cautioned against drawing conclusions about the numbers of deaths in these studies, the evidence suggests that safety has improved, not deteriorated."[255]

B. "Second, the report calls for more systematic approaches to the prevention of injuries due to medical care — for example, the use of computer systems to prevent such

---

[255] *Id.*

injuries…However, the systems are expensive to build, maintain, and upgrade. No health insurers or employers purchasing health insurance have been willing to pay for the extra expense."[256]

C. "Third, the IOM calls for a 50 percent reduction in the incidence of errors. This will be difficult to accomplish for several reasons… [N]o one has yet measured the incidence of errors in a general medical population. Without this important base-line information, it is impossible to document such a reduction, even if it is achievable."[257]

D. "Fourth, the publicity surrounding the IOM findings may lead to new reporting requirements. The IOM

---

[256] *Id.*
[257] *Id.*

recommends confidential, voluntary reporting of injuries due to medical care…Why, some might ask, should the public not know about blunders made by doctors? The answer is that most injuries from medical care are not due to mistakes…In addition, public disclosure would spawn lawsuits, which would in turn chill any interest in voluntary reporting."[258]

While we submit that these criticisms are fairly devastating, you may now be inquiring about the more recent papers we mentioned that offer even more grievous figures relating to medically caused deaths.

Dr. Kaveh G. Shojania and Professor Mary Dixon-Woods serve as editors of *British Medical Journal Quality and Safety*. They tackled the projections made by the "To Err Is Human" follow-ups in their paper "Estimating deaths due to medical error: the ongoing controversy and why it matters."[259] What they found were

---

[258] *Id.*

the same sorts of mistakes recycled into higher mortality projections.

Again, the studies did nothing in the way of a credible analysis of what sort of medical error might have actually been connected to a patient's death. They use the example of a patient admitted to an ICU for multisystem organ failure. Such a patient might develop a small rash from a minor allergic reaction to an antibiotic. This is certainly a preventable adverse event. If the patient dies, though, it is hardly fair to say that they expired due to the antibiotic they received.[260] Both papers, they point out, confound the issue of patients having a condition (say, a hospital-acquired infection) with a patient dying of a condition. Patients in danger of death are oftentimes more susceptible to infection. This type of mistake therefore "makes it very hard to allocate aliquots of blame to failures of medical management versus the patient's underlying illnesses. Thus, when errors are followed by death, it is only rarely straightforward to adjudicate the extent to which error contributed to death."[261]

---

[259] https://qualitysafety.bmj.com/content/26/5/423
[260] *Id.*
[261] *Id.*

Dr. Shojania and Prof. Woods also point out problems with the sample size used by the papers in question:

> For instance, one study used a trigger tool approach to review 100 charts per quarter from each of 10 hospitals in North Carolina from January 2002 to December 2007. This study sought to detect any decline in adverse events that might have occurred as a result of patient safety efforts. In passing, the authors report that 14 adverse events were judged to have 'caused or contributed to a patient's death'. These 14 deaths represented 0.6% of the total patients in the study. Similarly, one US government report included three preventable deaths; another reported 12. One of the widely quoted peer-reviewed studies identified nine deaths. Any extrapolation that generalises from so few deaths (14 or fewer) to so

many (200 000–400 000) surely warrants substantial scepticism.[262]

I have no doubt whatsoever that modern policy-makers reading this section will launch all sorts of invectives against it, probably by claiming that those making these points don't really care about patient safety and are clearly bad people who are okay with hundreds of thousands of patients dying from medical errors every year. These are, of course, very stupid accusations; however, we live in a time where stupid accusations can often get a lot of traction.

Really, though, all that is being proposed here is honesty, which is why the modern policy-maker will find it dangerous. The sorts of viscerally repulsive statistics cited by "To Err Is Human" and others strike a nerve with a lot of people. This makes them very useful for driving policy changes that fit the terms of The Compromise. Nobody can be bothered with whether or not the statistics in question are accurate. They are not important because they are accurate. They are important because they provide a means to an end.

Meanwhile, the end is realized more and more every day, as millions upon millions of dollars in

---

[262] *Id.*

regulatory actions are imposed upon providers under the semantic disguises of "value," "quality," and "patient safety." And is compliance with these measures praised or rewarded?

No, not really. "To Err is Human" has actually been made into a documentary film. Hospitals and physicians are still demonized as being at the root of all our health care problems, as should be obvious from the foregoing material in this book.

Regardless, even if one would like to argue that there is an enormous patient safety problem and that over half of all hospital deaths are somehow preventable, a reasonable approach would acknowledge the fact that there are so many credible critiques of the issue and that we should at least engage in greater study before diving headlong into proposed remedies that rely on such flimsy premises and distract us from taking actions that might potentially offer real benefits.

What about solutions, then? Are there any?

As long as all the relevant parties (payers, policy-makers, and patients) remain committed to The Compromise, the answer is no.

Chapter 13: What Will Solve All Of This(?)

I mentioned early on that I would not be offering much in the way of solutions. My goal here has primarily been to describe the problem as it actually is since most of the current popular ideas about what is wrong with healthcare are not backed up by reality.

I have proposed an alliance of interests between policy-makers, payers, and patients with Death itself. In the case of public officials/contractors and payers, this is a formal, strategic undertaking, largely focused on killing off patients' access to treatment. By doing so, they create a more secure budget or a stronger profit margin. For patients, their agreement to The Compromise is largely informal, being founded not on profits, but rather on the notion of convenience and entitlement. Actually changing healthcare is going to require one of these parties to break faith in The Compromise and embark on an honest and dedicated path to making things better.

Is this likely to happen in the case of payers? No. There are billions of dollars being made in selling insurance policies, taking over provider practices, and sifting patient data. What is their incentive to change? What money is there in actually approving and facilitating treatment for patients? All this does is create claims, which they then have to pay. The only access points payers wish to create are those that they own and manage, which allows for ultimate control over any patient options for care. With the ongoing takeover of Medicare and Medicaid by private payers, we see there being less and less chance for any grassroots movement or outrage to move the payers towards a more generous application of benefits.

They will always take the path of least resistance, and that path always means suppressing treatment for patients.

Are policy-makers any different? First, let's recall that policy-makers have been more than eager to pass the control of healthcare over to private payers as part of the aforementioned takeover of Medicare and Medicaid. This alone indicates some shared goals on their part.

Second, consider just the few regulatory schemes mentioned herein. Likewise, reflect on how they are imposed with a dearth of evidence to support them, in a one-size-fits-all manner, and with almost no focus on items that would actually improve a patient's health. Moreover, as we've seen, the outcomes of such regulatory burdens are typically negative in terms of providing good patient care. With all these things in mind, we must ask why our officials and their think-tank colleagues are constantly doubling down on such measures.

I'm very familiar with the warning not to mistake for malice what can be attributed to stupidity or to confuse correlation with causation. Are we not beyond this by now, though? We have admissions like those of Mr. Gruber in the Introduction. We have evidence that the current approach is not working to make people healthier, though it is working to destroy access to care. We have mobs of experts with Master's Degrees and PhDs all of whom claim this is the area of their expertise, and all of whom claim that this is the road to a better healthcare system. You can call this behavior whatever you like, from technocratic to sociopathic, but in my opinion, we are past calling it stupid. Regardless of the adjective you use, the failure to understand the behavior as intentional is a large part of what enables it to endure.[263]

Third, with the current mix of public policies in health care, efficiency means less and less. Rural hospitals are perhaps a canary in the coal mine to show what will

---

[263] Let me say here that, even if you choose to continue to think of the actions we've discussed as stupidity, I hope that you have still benefited from the book in the sense that you better understand the problems outlined.

happen to providers in the near future. Despite evidence that rural hospitals are "efficient, safe, and a lot cheaper"[264], they are closing down at a record pace since 2010. As I'm writing this, 120 have shuttered in that timeframe, with nearly 700 more labeled as financially "vulnerable" in a 2016 iVantage study. Still, even as efficient operators in a health care setting where the patients are disproportionately older, poorer, and sicker,[265] it is getting more and more difficult to carry on:

> "Being a CEO of a rural hospital today feels a bit like being Atlas in Greek mythology — the harder we strive to keep the doors open, the more regulatory and reimbursement weight is added," commented Leslie Marsh, CEO of Lexington Regional Health Center in Lexington, Nebraska. "The current financial and regulatory environment makes it very difficult

---

[264] https://www.healthcaredive.com/news/rural-health-care-efficient-safe-and-a-lot-cheaper/260313/; See also https://www.fiercehealthcare.com/healthcare/rural-hospitals-equal-outcomes-ahead-ed-care

[265] It's also more likely for such patients' care to be paid for by Medicare and Medicaid.

for small hospitals to remain profitable."[266]

These closures have an undeniable impact on their populations, with mortality increasing almost 6% in areas with a rural hospital closure.[267] There is also the added effect that a closed rural hospital usually destroys the economy of a rural community as well, increasing all of the negative social determinants of health as well.

All this being said, there are no meaningful initiatives to either salvage the rural safety net or to adopt rural models of care as examples of efficiency. Instead, we see the continued adoption of more and more burdens that take money away from patient care and raise fixed costs without any accompanying increases in payment.[268] The biggest avenue open to rural hospitals for survival is to be bought out or otherwise affiliating with a larger

---

[266] https://www.geneseorepublic.com/opinion/20191105/rural-hospitals---and-patients---are-at-risk
[267] https://www.beckershospitalreview.com/quality/rural-hospital-closures-increase-mortality-rates-study-finds.html
[268] On a side note, I know that many will simply try to write off rural hospital closures as being the result of population decline and unrelated to deliberate policy measures. I respond by asking, "Did rural populations suddenly reach some sort of critical mass in 2010 that caused all of these closures?" Populations have been decreasing for some time. Closures are recent. Any attempt to disconnect these closures from Medicare sequestration, EMR requirements, "value" and "quality" reporting, etc., is naïve at best and deceitful at worst.

healthcare system. Recent data shows that these steps improve the hospital's financial performance but still result in a loss of access to services for the community, albeit less severe than an outright closure.[269]

Finally, it is undeniable that the major cost differentiation between the US and other countries is the administrative costs.[270] Where do these administrative costs come from? From policy-makers and payers, who are the first groups to line up and proclaim that the solution to higher healthcare costs are more administrative burdens (i.e. costs).

Contemplating these factors, I cannot see any hope of the political/bureaucratic/consulting class doing anything other than what they are doing now. They will continue to drive providers out of the healthcare market by breaking them financially or burning them out.[271]

---

[269] https://revcycleintelligence.com/news/affiliation-boosts-rural-hospital-margins-but-reduces-care-access. This naturally carries with it the same potential problems with merger and acquisition mentioned in Chapter 10.

[270] https://www.nytimes.com/2018/07/16/upshot/costs-health-care-us.html. The other major drivers are labor and drug costs, see https://www.healthcaredive.com/news/labor-administrative-costs-drive-us-healthcare-spending-far-beyond-other-n/518994/

[271] https://www.healthexec.com/topics/policy/healthcare-providers-say-regulatory-burdens-are-rising

This brings us to the only member of The Compromise with any glimmer of hope at all. That would be us, the patients. Telling Americans that they are part of a problem is an unpopular thing. It's why nobody in Congress wants to do it. People have a natural tendency to reject an accusation of bad behavior on their part. Still, if the shoe fits…

The best public treatment I've seen of this matter is an article by David Freedman in the July 2019 edition of *The Atlantic*. The article is appropriately entitled "The Worst Patients In the World."[272] While I don't agree with 100% of Mr. Freedman's analysis, the overall theme and most of the specifics are correct. He summarizes all of the patient conduct issues that we have mentioned to this point. We don't take our medicine or comply with physician orders. We ignore our follow-ups. We demand treatments that are likely to be superfluous and reject others that require too much effort on our part. We then threaten our providers with legal action if the outcome is anything other than ideal.

He quotes one physician (who inadvertently makes the link with The Compromise) as saying, "We

<hr>

[272]

https://www.theatlantic.com/magazine/archive/2019/07/american-health-care-spending/590623/

tend to see health as something that policy making or health-care systems ought to do for us."

In other words, we participate in The Compromise not out of any financial gains but out of the need for convenience and the short-term gratification of doing what we please. Somebody else will take action to make us healthy. We think that our being well is something that will happen because Congress passed a law, a hospital expanded its services, a drug company came out with a new medication, or some other external intervention. As previously discussed, 40% of our health is governed by individual behaviors and choices. Payers and policy-makers, being all-in on The Compromise, take advantage of our bad ones.[273]

The only thing that can improve healthcare, then, is for us to take better care of ourselves. At a time when obesity-related illnesses such as diabetes and heart disease run rampant, taking the time to engage in our personal well-being is the best we can do. We cannot simply look for a clinician to offer us a pill for our problems.[274] We

---

[273] I take for granted that we can't do anything about genetics and are probably limited in how we can address social/environmental factors.

[274] Consider the incoherence, for example, of those who bemoan the enormous influence of drug companies in American healthcare yet simultaneously demand for all of their problems to be resolved by a

cannot look for the convenient or easy solution for what ails us. Even in the existence of so-called "food deserts," the mere act of walking and eschewing the couch and television would show vast improvements.[275] Naturally, it would be equally wonderful to heed our physician's instructions (while we can still see a physician) on other types of behavior, take our medicines appropriately, and avoid whatever negative environmental factors we can. I'm just starting with the simple things.

Do I think this will happen?

No.

Speaking as an awful and non-compliant patient myself, I understand the intense inertia that surrounds any sort of lifestyle change, regardless of how minor. We tell ourselves that we don't have the time, the place, or the circumstances to allow for such changes. When faced with the decision to take a 30 minute walk or binge watch on the new streaming channel, we take the path of least resistance.

From 2014-2017, life expectancy in the US decreased. This is primarily attributed to increasing deaths

---

miracle drug (assuming they take it as instructed in the first place).
[275] https://www.nbcnews.com/better/health/why-walking-most-underrated-form-exercise-ncna797271

among working age adults.[276] When the specifics behind these deaths are observed, many tend to have a common root in person behaviors:

> Specifically, deaths in midlife adults increased by:
>
> - 386.5% from drug overdoses
> - 40.6% from alcoholic liver disease
> - 78.9% from hypertension
> - 114.0% from obesity
>
> In particular age groups, things were much worse. In adults aged 25 to 34 years, deaths from alcoholic liver disease increased 157.6%. Adults aged 55 to 64 years had a 909.2% increase in overdose deaths…[277]

Patients must begin to reject those sorts of behaviors if we are to see any improvements in the healthcare system overall.

---

[276] https://jamanetwork.com/journals/jama/fullarticle/2756187
[277] https://www.mdlinx.com/internal-medicine/article/5501

More than that, the existence of smartphones, online shopping, Wi-Fi, etc. are feeding our societal drive for convenience over real service. Even in healthcare, we see online "doctor on demand" services where patients simply link up to a physician for a "virtual visit" on their smartphone, allow the physician to diagnose them, and then even prescribe them medication all over a phone camera. This physician has not laid hands on this patient, has not taken a single vital sign, and is 100% reliant on the patient's personal recollection of their medical history. Solely out of convenience, though, this patient will accept "treatment" during such an encounter. How can this be regarded as good health care? This "consumerization," organizing care strictly for patient convenience, has become a huge arena of investment, banking entirely on the idea that consumer patients will take the quick and easy path, rather than something more thorough and more likely to help them. This, of course, assumes the patient even has the option of seeing a flesh and blood provider in their area at all.

Not only, then, are we fighting against our own human natures in order to do what is right for our health, those impulses that incline us to choose contrary to our well-being are being nurtured and cultivated by others.

Meanwhile, the clinicians who are still in the market to provide guidance and treatment for this patient population are being drained of their financial and emotional resources, all in the name of programs that, to this day, still show very little in the way of achieving their publicly stated goals.[278] We will eventually see them cast off these burdens and opt for cash-only transactions catering to well-off patients who are likely healthier and easier to care for.

I realize that this entire conclusion is very dark. I only promised honesty in this book and cannot manufacture faux sunshine here at the end just to close with a happy ending. Any good physician will tell you that treating a problem is a waste of time without a proper diagnosis. Getting to a proper diagnosis has been the focus of this endeavor. Others must formulate and implement the broader solutions. As a nation, though, we must each as individuals (a) recognize that our lives and health are being exchanged for budgets, profits, and

---

[278] I offer one final example under the caption of "Value-based pay still struggles to improve costs, quality" taken from https://www.modernhealthcare.com/payment/value-based-pay-still-struggles-improve-costs-quality. Even with more than half of commercial payments being tied to "value" and a growing percentage of Medicare payments doing likewise, with little benefit in sight, the concluding proposal is to shift still more risk onto the providers.

societal control; (b) recognize our own complicity in that exchange; and (c) after recognizing how we are complicit, eliminate those factors that make us so.

Until then, we are at the mercy of our healthcare overlords, and they will continue to deal us away as currency in The Reaper's Compromise.

Thank you for purchasing my book. If you found it to be an informative and worthwhile read, please consider leaving a review on Amazon, Goodreads, Facebook, or other platforms that you enjoy.

For continued news, updates, and commentary on healthcare matters, be sure to visit and subscribe to our website at www.thereaperscompromise.wordpress.com.